Toxicology of the Blood and Bone Marrow
Target Organ Toxicology Series

Target Organ Toxicology Series

Editor-in-Chief: Robert L. Dixon
U.S. EPA, Office of Health Effects, Washington, D.C.

Target Organ Toxicology Series

Toxicology of the Blood and Bone Marrow

Editor

Richard D. Irons, Ph.D.

Departments of Cell Biology, and Experimental Pathology and Toxicology
Chemical Industry Institute of Toxicology
Research Triangle Park, North Carolina

Raven Press ■ New York

Raven Press, 1140 Avenue of the Americas, New York, New York 10036

Made in the United States of America

Library of Congress Cataloging in Publication Data

Main entry under title:

Toxicology of the blood and bone marrow.

    (Target organ toxicology series)
    Includes bibliographies and index.
    1. Marrow—Diseases. 2. Blood—Diseases.
3. Toxicology. I. Irons, Richard D. II. Series.
[DNLM: 1. Blood Cells—drug effects. 2. Bone Marrow—
drug effects. QY 402 T755]
RC645.7.T69 1985   615'.718   85-1919
ISBN 0-89004-837-1

International Standard Book Number 0-89004-837-1
Library of Congress Catalog Card Number

To Beverly, Kati, David and Sarah

Preface

The blood and bone marrow constitute a widely dispersed organ system comprised of a heterogeneous population of cells that provide diverse functions to the host. Mature erythrocytes, granulocytes, macrophages, platelets and lymphocytes all have their origins in cells residing in the bone marrow and ultimately are derived from a single pluripotent stem cell. Hemopoiesis is dependent on the continuing self-renewal and differentiation of bone marrow stem cells. Toxicity to the blood and bone marrow can be manifested as a result of the destruction of mature cells, their precursor cells, impaired cell growth or differentiation. Traditionally, the toxicologist has evaluated potential toxicity to the blood and bone marrow by analyzing hemograms and assessing the numbers of circulating blood cells. The last two decades have witnessed a rapid growth in basic knowledge of the structure of cells that has contributed considerably to our understanding of the complexity and function of the hemopoietic system. These advances in experimental hematology have resulted in a recognition of the importance of studying bone marrow toxicity in terms of the structure and dynamics of hemopoiesis and have provided the toxicologist with a bewildering array of additional tools with which to approach the task.

Although written largely by specialists in experimental and clinical hematology, this volume is intended for toxicologists, pharmacologists and other scientists engaged in studying the effects of chemicals on the hemopoietic system. It was comissioned to provide a basic overview of hematology, to summarize the current status of experimentation in the field, and to introduce the reader to newer methods and approaches applicable to the study of blood and bone marrow toxicity. Subject areas include the development, structure and function of the bone marrow, regulation of hemopoiesis, toxicology of the erythrocyte and granulocyte, the use of stem cell assays, flow cytofluorometry and cytogenetic techniques for assessing bone marrow damage, the role of the bone marrow as a metabolic organ in the bioactivation of benzene, and occupational factors associated with chemically induced leukemia and lymphoma in man.

The expansion of research in hematology continues to provide increasingly sophisticated and sensitive approaches for the evaluation of chemical toxicity to the blood and bone marrow. It is hoped that their integration with other approaches in toxicology will form the basis for continued improvement in the prediction of human risk associated with exposure to myelotoxic agents.

Richard D. Irons

Foreword

The *Target Organ Toxicology* monographs have evolved from the need for periodic review of the methods used to assess chemically induced toxicity. In each monograph, experts focus upon the following areas of a particular organ system: (1) a review of the morphology, physiology, biochemistry, cellular biology, and developmental aspects of the system; (2) a description of the means routinely used to assess toxicity; (3) an evaluation of the feasibility of tests used in the assessment of hazards; (4) proposals for applying recent advances in the basic sciences to the development and validation of new test procedures; (5) a description of the incidence of chemically induced human disease; and (6) an assessment of the reliability of laboratory test data extrapolation to humans and of the methods currently used to estimate human risk.

Thus, these monographs should be useful to both students and professionals of toxicology. Each provides a concise description of organ toxicity, including an up-to-date review of the biological processes represented by the target organ, a summary of how chemicals perturb these processes and alter function, and a description of methods by which such toxicity is detected in laboratory animals and humans. Attention is also directed to the identification of probable toxic chemicals and the establishment of exposure standards which are both economically and scientifically feasible, while adequately protecting human health and the environment.

Robert L. Dixon
Editor-in-Chief

Contents

Contributors

Ernest Beutler
Scripps Clinic and Research Foundation
Department of Basic and Clinical
Research
Division of Hematology/Oncology
10666 North Torrey Pines Road
La Jolla, California 92037

I. Chanarin
Medical Research Council's Clinical
Research Centre
Northwick Park Hospital
Harrow, Middlesex, United Kingdom

Eugene P. Cronkite
Medical Research Center
Brookhaven National Laboratory
Upton, New York 11973

William F. Greenlee
Department of Cell Biology
Chemical Industry Institute of Toxicology
Research Triangle Park, North Carolina
27709

Richard D. Irons
Departments of Cell Biology, and
Experimental Pathology and
Toxicology
Chemical Industry Institute of Toxicology
Research Triangle Park, North Carolina
27709

J. L. Ivett
Litton Bionetics, Inc.,
5516 Nicholson Lane,
Kensington, Maryland 20895

John C. Marsh
Yale University School of Medicine
333 Cedar Street
New Haven, Connecticut 06510

Douglas E. Rickert
Department of General and Biochemical
Toxicology
Chemical Industry Institute of Toxicology
Research Triangle Park, North Carolina
27709

Tadashi Sawahata
Toxicology Laboratory
Toray Industries, Inc.
2-7-35 Sonoyama
Otsu 520, Japan

Wayne S. Stillman
Department of Cell Biology
Chemical Industry Institute of Toxicology
Research Triangle Park, North Carolina
27709

Raymond R. Tice
Medical Department
Brookhaven National Laboratory
Upton, New York 11973

Theodora A. Tsongas
Office of Standards Review
Health Standards Program
Occupational Safety and Health
Administration
U.S. Department of Labor
200 Constitution Avenue, N.W.
Washington, D.C. 20210

Floyd D. Wilson
U.S. Department of Agriculture
Western Regional Research Center
800 Buchanan Street
Berkeley, California 94710

Toxicology of the Blood and Bone Marrow, edited by Richard D. Irons. Raven Press, New York © 1985.

Structure and Function of the Bone Marrow

I. Chanarin

Medical Research Council's Clinical Research Centre, Northwick Park Hospital, Harrow, Middlesex, United Kingdom

In all species blood formation occurs in the marrow throughout life. The nature of hemopoiesis and the characteristics of bone marrow that enable it to provide a suitable environment for hemopoiesis is the subject of this chapter. Human marrow has always been difficult to study in depth, because of both the difficulty in obtaining material without trauma and the presence of bony trabeculae, which makes handling the material difficult. Most research has used mouse marrow where the central femur is without trabeculae so that material can be easily fixed after perfusion. Human marrow has not been studied using electron microscopy (EM) and related techniques in the way that has been the case with the mouse. There are differences but the basic mechanisms are the same.

In the human embryo hemopoiesis, detectable initially in the yolk sac after the 19th day of gestation, develops in the liver after the fifth week and in the marrow after the 20th week, where myeloid and megakaryocyte proliferation continue. Red cell production (erythropoiesis) remains restricted to fetal liver and spleen until the last trimester of pregnancy, and at term hemopoiesis in man is confined to the marrow. Pluripotential stem cells have been reported, using clonal assays, by the 12th week in human fetal liver and by the 15th week in marrow (17).

The marrow of the neonate is completely taken up by hemopoietic cells, and there is little possibility of expanding blood production into medullary sites in response to stress at this age. Fat starts to appear in bones of the terminal digits *in utero*, and at the end of the first year the bones of the toes are completely fatty. At the age of 4 years fat spaces in significant amount are present in the marrow cavity of long bones, and these normally expand until at the age of 18 years active hemopoiesis is present only in the central skeleton, that is, the vertebrae, ribs, pelvis, skull and proximal ends of the long bones. During hemopoietic stress with a requirement for increased blood formation, active hemopoiesis can return to these fatty areas.

In the adult some 4.6% of body weight is due to marrow and its mass in a 70-kg man has been estimated at 1,460 g. Thus, in size it is comparable to the liver.

BLOOD SUPPLY TO THE MARROW

Arterial blood reaches the marrow from two sources, the nutrient artery and small arteries derived from those supplying attached muscles. The nutrient artery passes through the cortex of the bone via the nutrient canal and in the medullary cavity divides into ascending and descending branches, which, in turn, give off smaller radial branches to the inner surface of the cortex. The cortical blood from both muscular arteries and radial branches enters the marrow from the endosteal surface of the cortex, branching and narrowing to capillaries approximately 4 μm in diameter, and leads to a complex branching of medullary sinuses, which in turn collect into a larger central sinus, and finally into the emissary vein passing through the nutrient canal to join the systemic venous circulation (Fig. 1).

THE HEMOPOIETIC MICROENVIRONMENT

The concept of a hemopoietic microenvironment is both a morphological one when referring to the elements in marrow that provide mechanical support for developing hemopoietic cells, and a functional one including the local factors that permit stem cells to develop along particular lines.

In normal animals the pluripotential hemopoietic stem cell circulates freely in peripheral blood, but it is only in the marrow that these cells are able to develop into mature blood cells. Thus the hemopoietic microenvironment must involve sites that are able to recognize and retain stem cells. Similarly in irradiated animals reconstituted with donor marrow cells, hemopoietic colonies develop only in marrow and in some species in the spleen (49), but in no other tissues. The development of extramedullary hemopoiesis is always preceded by the appearance of marrow vasculature and stroma at the site. Thus, marrow fibroblasts (but not fibroblasts from elsewhere) when transplanted beneath the renal capsule give rise to a stromal

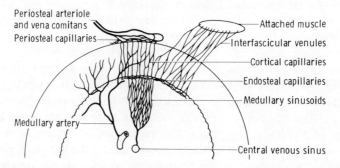

FIG. 1. The nutrient artery passes through the cortex and bifurcates in the marrow cavity into ascending and descending medullary branches from which radial arteries pass to the inner surface of the cortex. Periosteal blood reaches bone through the arteries of attached muscles and periosteal and endosteal capillaries communicate. The cortical capillaries enter the marrow sinuses, which collect into the central venous sinuses, and these join the emissary vein, which drains blood from the bone. [Reproduced with permission from Brooke, M. (1971): *The Blood Supply of Bone*, Butterworth, London.]

structure which in turn becomes populated by hemopoietic cells (47). These observations imply that certain tissues provide a microenvironment that alone has the capacity to support hemopoiesis. Marrow fragments transplanted to extramedullary sites rapidly lose their hemopoietic cells. Stromal elements proliferate, however, and when this is established, repopulation by hemopoietic cells occurs (14). Radiation in excess of 1,500 R destroys marrow stroma and stem cells and is irreversible. But curettage of marrow is reversible with return of stroma followed later by return of hemopoiesis (32).

Studies in the mechanism of congenital macrocytic anemias in mice bear out these concepts. Mice with the Steel anemia (Sl/Sl^d) have normal pluripotential hemopoietic stem cells but are stroma deficient. Wv/Wv mice have an anemia due to absence of functional stem cells. Splenic tissue from Wv/Wv mice, by supplying stromal cells, can cure the anemia of Sl/Sl^d mice. Marrow from stromal-deficient Sl/Sl^d mice can protect recipient animals from the lethal effects of radiation, confirming that they have their own pluripotential hemopoietic stem cells.

Cellulose acetate membranes coated with macrophages and fibroblasts from marrow and spleen, when implanted into the peritoneal cavities of lethally irradiated animals given donor marrow cells, become the site of hemopoiesis in these animals (20).

Long-term culture of marrow stem cells provides the *in vitro* equivalent of this situation. Establishment of long-term culture requires the establishment of a culture of marrow-derived adherent cells. This adherent layer consists of endothelial-like cells, fat cells, and macrophages. Once such a stromal layer is established, hemopoietic cells will grow and renew themselves in this environment.

It proved impossible to establish such long-term cultures from Sl/Sl^d or Wv/Wv mice. But when an adherent layer was produced from Wv/Wv mice, hemopoietic cell growth from Sl/Sl^d mice was achieved. It was not possible to produce an adherent layer from Sl/Sl^d mice that apparently lack stromal cells (11).

THE MICROSCOPIC STRUCTURE OF THE MARROW

The Venous Sinuses

Marrow contains an elaborate system of thin-walled, branching, anastomosing venous vessels called the venous sinuses. They are 15 to 100 μm in diameter, and the wall consists of three layers—the endothelium, the basement membrane, and the adventitia. A further cell, the adventitial reticular cell, is associated with the adventitia. Hemopoietic cells are situated immediately outside the sinus wall, and the mature blood cells traverse the wall of the venous sinus to enter the circulation.

Endothelium cells line the inner surface of the venous sinus completely. Like all endothelial cells, they are broad and flat with irregular loosely overlapping cytoplasmic edges. Their nuclei may protrude into the lumen or outward. Holes develop readily in the endothelium to allow passage of mature blood cells, although most holes seen in preparations are artifacts. The endothelium also contains transcytotic vesicles, microfilaments, microtubules, some mitochondria, and lysosomes. Endocytosis allows materials from the blood to traverse the endothelial cell. The endothelial cell, too, can be phagocytic (22,52,53). A basement membrane comprising a carbohydrate-protein complex similar to that in reticular fibers is present. Endothelial cells have been reported to produce burst-promoting activity (BPA) required for erythropoiesis (54).

Adventitial Reticular Cell

These cells line the adventitial surface of the venous sinuses and form part of the adventitial coat. They have extensive, broad, cytoplasmic processes that may cover about one- to two-thirds of the sinus surface. The reticular cells synthesize argentiphilic fibers that may be identical with collagen types I and III (3). They show variable expression of factor VIII-associated antigen, synthesize proteoglycans, and express the common acute lymphoblastic leukemia antigen. However, they lack an antigen (T-200) present on all other hemopoietic cells. Using long-term culture of human marrow, Singer et al. (43) showed that what is presumably the adventitial reticular cell (marrow stromal cell) arose from the same pluripotential stem cell that gave rise to all the other hemopoietic cells.

The reticular cell is capable of considerable changes in volume with uncovering of the sinus surface, which may possibly aid egress of mature hemopoietic cells. The adventitial reticular cells not only are in contact with the venous sinuses but are also in direct contact with developing hemopoietic cells, and the reticular fibrils constitute part of the marrow stroma providing the hemopoietic microenvironment. The adventitial cells may also become fatty and so become the adipocytes of marrow.

The adventitial reticular cell may also be the marrow fibroblast. Such fibroblasts, when explanted out of the marrow, give rise to hemopoietic stroma and can form bone. In this respect they differ from fibroblasts of other sources, which too are present in marrow, including adventitial cells of marrow arteries, bone-associated cells, and cells lining nerve sheaths. The cytoplasmic processes extending from the reticular cells not only surround the venous sinus but also extend out from one sinus to another, providing an intersinus, extravascular network. These reticular processes are intimately related to granulopoiesis, and these cells may produce granulocyte-monocyte growth factor (7,39). The role of such cells in long-term marrow culture has been discussed.

ADIPOCYTES (FAT CELLS)

The fat cells of marrow differ in many respects from fat cells in other tissues. Marrow fat cells are less affected by dietary restrictions that induce lipolysis in fat stores elsewhere (2,44). The fat in marrow cells is unsaturated whereas that elsewhere is essentially saturated, and marrow fat has a different fatty acid composition (45,50). Fat-cell formation in marrow is not promoted by insulin, unlike the situation in other tissues (16). They lack glycogen and have reduced endoplasmic reticulum during lipid synthesis. Marrow fat cells convert androgens to estrogens (15) and induce granulopoiesis in long-term cultures. Developing clusters of granulocytes adhere tightly to cells undergoing reticular cell-adipocyte transformation.

The origin of marrow adipocytes is likely to be the adventitial reticular cell, and their frequent location outside the venous sinusoid favors this origin. Marrow adipocytes can transform into fibroblasts in culture (30) by lipolysis of the fat. Within the marrow the adipocytes occupy space not required for hemopoiesis.

NERVE TISSUE

Myelinated and nonmyelinated nerve fibers accompany vessels in marrow, and Schwann cells are present. They probably regulate arterial wall tone.

MACROPHAGES

Macrophages are an important constituent of the hemopoietic microenvironment. In marrow they are found within erythroblastic islands, within lymphoblastic islets, in close association with developing eosinophils and other leukocytes, closely applied to vascular sinuses, and, occasionally, free within the lumen of a sinus. Hudson and Shortland (19) suggested that the adventitial reticular cell is a modified macrophage and this would be compatible with its origin from the pluripotential hemopoietic stem cell. The macrophage may have several functions to play in the marrow. Phagocytosis is important and includes ingestion of defective erythroblasts (ineffective hemopoiesis), extruded erythroblast nuclei during erythroblast maturation, perhaps of surplus iron-containing particles, ingestion in lymphoblast islets of imperfect cells or expressing forbidden clones, and so on. Macrophages on the outside surface of venous sinus may exercise surveillance over passage of materials to and from vessels. Macrophages in several species have been shown to extend pseudopodia into the venous sinus and to ingest circulating (? senescent) red cells (46), but there is increasing evidence that the role of the macrophage is more significant than that of phagocytosis. They may stimulate granulopoiesis by elaborating colony-stimulating factor and influence erythropoiesis by producing BPA (36). Acidic isoferritins present in macrophages may regulate granulopoiesis (5,6). Bessis (4) drew attention to the intimate relation between the macrophage and erythropoiesis in marrow, and the manner in which the protrusion of macrophage cytoplasm surrounds each cell in an erythroblast island is shown in Fig. 2, which was drawn from an EM photograph (52). The most immature cells lie in the center and the more mature to the periphery of the island. Isolated erythroblasts in marrow are unusual. Proerythroblasts and erythroblasts show extensive regions of intimate membrane contact with the central macrophage over large areas of their surface, but this association is reduced in the reticulocyte. Gap junctions between the macrophage and early erythroblasts have been reported. "Coated pits" in the erythroblast membrane at areas closely apposed to the macrophage have been noted, and these can serve as transport organelles carrying receptor-bound protein, such as receptor-bound transferrin iron, into cells (1).

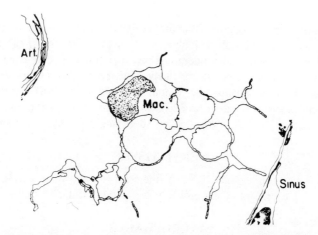

FIG. 2. Tracing of a single macrophage (Mac) extending long, slender, branching processes that enclose erythroblasts in different degrees of maturation in an erythroblast island. The venous sinus and an artery are marked. In preparation the marrow had been perfused before fixation, and this led to separation of the constituent cells. (Reproduced with permission from Weiss, ref. 52.)

LYMPHOCYTES

Like macrophages, lymphocytes appear to be associated with maturation of all hemopoietic cell lines. Their physical relationship to developing cell lines is less clear than with macrophages. They may be in contact with hemopoietic cells or separated from them. Presumably the effect of lymphocytes is mediated by release of humoral substances. The effect has been best characterized in the requirement for T-helper cells in erythropoiesis (31), an effect produced in tandem with macrophages (36).

LOCATION OF HEMOPOIESIS

Erythroblastic clusters are closer than granulocytic clusters to the venous sinuses. Late erythroblasts and metamyelocytes lie near the sinus wall whereas the earlier stages are deeper in the hemopoietic tissues. Hemopoiesis is most active near bone. Megakaryocytes are located on the surface of the venous sinusoids, undergoing polyploidy and discharging platelets through apertures in the sinus well into the circulation.

HEMOPOIESIS

The Pluripotential Stem Cell

It is now established that a common stem cell gives rise to erythrocytes, granulocytes, monocytes, macrophages and their derivatives, platelets, and B and T lymphocytes. The evidence is the presence of chromosomal mutation of single-cell origin in all those hemopoietic cells. This occurs in chronic myeloid leukemia and is best demonstrated in patients heterozygous for glucose-6-phosphate dehydrogenase (G6PD). This enzyme is carried on the X-chromosome, and as in each cell, one of the X-chromosomes is normally suppressed; in a person inheriting an A variant and a B variant of G6PD, the cells will be an equal mixture of A and B variants. Patients with chronic myeloid leukemia have a characteristic translocation of part of chromosome 22 to chromosome 9. Hemopoietic cells in chronic myeloid leukemia carry only the B variant of G6PD, or the A variant whereas other cells, such as the skin, have the expected mixture of A and B variants. This combination of translocated chromosome and a single enzyme variant is present in all hemopoietic cell lines, indicating that they are all the progeny of a mutation of a single pluripotential stem cell. Thus the pluripotential stem cell gives rise to all hemopoietic cells.

The stem cell has two attributes: It will maintain its own numbers by self-renewal, and under appropriate stimulation it differentiates into mature functional cells.

Basic understanding of stem cell behavior has come from mouse studies. In the mouse the spleen is an important hemopoietic organ. Rescue of the irradiated mouse with donor marrow cells is accompanied by the appearance of discrete modules of hemopoietic cells in the spleen. Each module arises from a single pluripotential stem cell. This has provided a means of stem cell assay. The cell that is able to produce a colony has been termed spleen colony-forming cell (CFC-S).

In other species such an assay is not available, and in man an *in vitro* assay has been developed in either agar or methylcellulose in the presence of an extract from normal peripheral blood leukocytes grown in the presence of phytohemagglutinin (24). The colonies that develop arise from a single inoculated cell, and they may contain erythroid, myeloid, and megakaryocytic elements, implying origin from a pluripotential stem cell. Such cells have been termed colony-forming unit-granulocyte, erythroid, macrophage, megakaryocyte (CFU-GEMM). It is clear, however, that such an assay underestimates stem cell numbers. Human marrows treated with 4-hydroperoxycyclophosphamide produce few CFU-GEMM colonies, but when given to patients whose marrows have been ablated, marrow reconstitution has occurred (40). Alternatively, CFU-GEMM is not the pluripotential stem cell.

Similar observations have emerged with CFU-S in the mouse. When a mouse is reconstituted with normal marrow following a dose of lethal irradiation, the CFU-S in the reconstituted mouse has a reduced capacity to rescue another mouse treated in the same way, that is, there has been a reduction in the capacity of the stem cell for self-renewal. The same applies to man given high-dose irradiation or cytotoxic therapy and rescued with return of autologous-stored marrow. When the process is repeated a second time with marrow collected and stored between treatments, there is delayed reconstitution. This has given rise to the suggestion that the stem cell is a fixed cell in "niches" within the hemopoietic microenvironment where it is protected but can be stimulated to become the cell recognized as CFU-S or CFU-GEMM.

Studies with the "thymidine-suicide" technique, where a large dose of [³H]thymidine will kill those dividing cells that take it up, suggest that in the mouse approximately 10% of CFU-S are "active" so that the bulk are resting cells (41).

In man hemopoietic progenitor cells can be isolated from peripheral blood in the null mononuclear cell fraction, that is, in the cells remaining after polymorphs, T and B lymphocytes, and macrophages have been removed. They can be concentrated effectively from peripheral blood on cell separators when the concentrations compare favorably with those present in marrow (21).

Apart from sensitivity to irradiation, CFU-S is killed by busulfan used in the treatment of chronic myeloid leukemia, and temporary damage is produced by isopropylmethane sulfonate.

Pluripotential hemopoietic stem cells are recognized by their behavior in test systems. Their morphological recognition has not been achieved.

Erythroid Progenitor Cells

The earliest identifiable red cell precursor in marrow is the proerythroblast. Before this stage, red cell precursors undergo a series of divisions from the pluripotential stem cell, which are identified only by clonal assays. These stages have been identified in man as well as in the mouse (48).

Burst-Forming Unit-Erythroid (BFU-E)

Marrow or null cells derived from peripheral blood give rise to large multiple hemoglobinized colonies on methylcellulose or plasma clot cultures after 10 to 14 days' incubation. It may contain a few hundred to ten thousand erythroblasts. The early cells in this colony are mobile, and hence migrate, to give the characteristic appearance. The larger colonies are visible to the naked eye. Each colony arises from a single cell as assessed by the glucose-6-phosphate isoenzyme type (35).

Colony-Forming Unit-Erythroid (CFU-E)

Marrow cells from man when plated out on methylcellulose show small colonies appearing after approximately 5 to 7 days. These do not develop further and presumably arise from a precursor that is nearer the proerythroblast than the BFU-E. In the mouse these colonies appear in 1 to 3 days.

Factors Influencing Erythroid Progenitor Cells

The development of erythroid precursors requires the presence of a hormone erythropoietin and the presence of macrophage and T-helper lymphocytes, which also may function through the secretion of stimulatory or inhibitory substances.

The development of BFU-E in the early stages does not require erythropoietin but requires a factor present in serum. Its early growth is promoted by the presence of small numbers of macrophages, but in larger numbers macrophages are inhibitory to growth. The factor stimulating development of BFU-E has been termed burst-promoting activity (BPA). It has been suggested that monocytes also produce a factor that stimulates BPA production in endothelial cell culture (54). Hemin augments the growth of BFU-E in culture (28).

T-helper lymphocytes are also required for optimal development of BFU-E (31). Erythroid cell cultures require the addition of erythropoietin, but this can be added after a few days incubation without affecting the outcome, implying that it acts at a later stage of development. The cells appearing in the presence of macrophages alone may derive from a more primitive progenitor than those appearing after lymphocytes are added. The early colonies are megaloblastic in morphology and still synthesize fetal hemoglobin (HbF) whereas those grown in the presence of T cells are normoblastic with lower levels of fetal hemoglobin (38). Although it has been suggested that a T-cell requirement is present only with peripheral blood stem cells, this can be shown for marrow cells if sufficient care is taken to remove macrophages (23,37). In the clinical situation patients with chronic lymphatic leukemia involving mainly T-suppressor cells may have anemia due to failure of erythropoiesis alone, but it has proved very difficult to demonstrate that the T-suppressor cells have such an effect on *in vitro* cell culture systems. The T-suppressor cell may well have a role in erythropoiesis, but this has yet to be demonstrated.

Erythropoietin

This is a glycoprotein hormone produced largely in the kidney, but there is probably a small contribution from the liver. It is found in high levels in serum and urine of anemic individuals, the only exception being anemia accompanying severe renal disease. In culture of erythroid progenitors in the absence of erythropoietin, cell division continues, but only when erythropoietin is added is there differentiation into and amplification of cells into proerythroblasts.

Recently several groups developed radioimmunoassays for erythropoietin that will supplant the cumbersome *in vivo* assays (10), but the scarcity of purified erythropoietin remains an obstacle to further development.

Granulocyte Monocyte Progenitors

Granulocyte progenitors can be induced to produce colonies in soft agar culture when they are incubated with colony-stimulating factor (CSF). This is sometimes called granulocyte-macrophage colony stimulating factor (GM-CSF) or eosinophil colony-stimulating factor (EO-CSF) in case of eosinophils. The source of GM-CSF is either peripheral blood leukocytes used as an underlayer in culture (25,34), phytohemagglutinin-stimulated T lymphocytes, or human placenta. The source of progenitor cells is marrow or peripheral blood. Mouse cultures are read after 7 days incubation at 37°C in 7.5% CO_2 and human cultures read after 10 to 14 days or even later (13). The colony numbers are scored by placing the petri dish on a grid and scanning the colonies, which are composed of 40 to several thousand cells. They may be picked off and stained, and 20% to 30% will be found to be eosinophil. There are marked differences in the appearance and development of individual colonies in the same culture. Adjacent colonies may be composed entirely of myeloblasts or myelocytes, polymorphs, monocytes, or mixtures of all four. A single committed cell generates both monocytes and neutrophil polymorphs.

The CSF appears to be a glycoprotein. Other putative regulators include prostaglandins (inhibiting GM-CSF production), lactoferrin, and a granulocyte chalone (9). The CSFs are of varying molecular weight ranging from 23,000, 45,000, and 65,000 and may be composed of a polymer of subunits (29). There may be separate factors for stimulating neutrophils, macrophages, as well as eosinophils. The macrophage may be a source of both CSF, prostaglandin, and lactoferrin. The last is also produced by granulocytes.

Lymphoid Progenitors

T and B lymphocytes arise from the pluripotential hemopoietic stem cell in the marrow. A T-cell line may separate at a very early stage of maturation, since chromosomal abnormalities in leukemia have been noted in erythroid, myeloid, megakaryocytic, and B-lymphocyte lines that have, however, spared the T lymphocytes. Both T and B lymphocytes may be lacking in combined immunodeficiency in man, although the implication of this is less clear. These early cells are believed to be 3 or 4 cell divisions away from cells recognizably committed to lymphoid differentiation. The marrow is the primary site in man for the production of B lymphocytes. T cells arise initially in the marrow from the pluripotential stem cell (prethymocytes), but thereafter the vast majority of T cells derive from the thymus gland, where the prethymocytes, under the influence of thymosin, become postthymic T cells.

The clonal growth of lymphoid colonies from early progenitors is at a relatively early stage of development, but colonies in agar have been produced for both T and B cells, as has growth in long-term culture (27,42).

Megakaryocytic Progenitors

The origin of megakaryocytes from the pluripotential hemopoietic stem cell is well established. Cytotoxic agents that depress other hemopoietic cell lines tend to have a delayed effect on reducing platelet levels. The mature platelet-producing megakaryocytes are not in cell cycle, and the nonplatelet-producing precursors are affected. This is a nonpolyploid-(2N) committed progenitor cell compartment that may be in a state of rest and that is able to respond to stimuli for platelet production (12).

Clonogenic assays with marrow cells detect CFU-MK in culture. Committed precursors occur in peripheral blood (18). There is a feedback control system. Acute thrombocytopenia causes an increase in size, DNA content, and number of megakaryocytes maturing; transfusion-induced thrombocytosis has the reverse effect. Regulation is probably mediated by a humoral substance termed thrombopoietin, which appears to be present in plasma. It has been suggested that

megakaryocyte-stimulating factor (MK-CSA) acts on early progenitors and thrombopoietin on later ones (33).

In hemopoietic arrest, usually due to infection with a parvovirus, young, single
nuclear megakaryocytes (so-called giant proerythroblasts) appear in the marrow 4
to 5 days after the start of the episode and are followed by a rise in the platelet
count on day 6 (8). The time probably reflects the time sequence from pluripotential
cell to platelet-producing megakaryocyte. The corresponding time with erythroblast
development is 10 days.

Morphology of Human Bone Marrow

Progenitor cells are not recognized in stained preparation of marrow since their
numbers are too low. Their progeny are present in normal marrow. Normal marrow
is a mixture of fat cells and intervening areas of hemopoiesis. A hypoplastic or
aplastic sample is largely composed of fat, with few hemopoietic cells, and in a
hypercellular sample there is an increase in hemopoietic cells, owing to increased
blood regeneration, at the expense of fat spaces, which may largely disappear. The
description that follows applies to marrow spreads properly fixed in anhydrous
methyl alcohol and stained by a Romanowsky method.

Erythropoiesis

The earliest recognizable cell is the proerythroblast, which is a large round cell
(18 μ diameter), a large nucleus of finely divided chromatin, and often one or
more nucleoli. The thin rim of cytoplasm is deeply basophilic, often with a
perinuclear clear zone. Maturation and further cell division lead to loss of nucleoli
and the cell is termed a basophilic erythroblast (or basophilic normoblast). Thereafter the nucleus becomes smaller, as does the cell, and the synthesis of hemoglobin
results in the cytoplasm taking on a grey instead of a deep blue coloration. This is
termed a polychromatic erythroblast. Finally the nucleus becomes pyknotic and the
cytoplasm pink. At this stage the nucleus is extruded. The erythrocyte still contains
RNA, which will precipitate with dyes such as brilliant cresyl blue, enabling one
to recognize these young cells, which are termed reticulocytes. They remain in the
marrow for 1 to 2 days and are then released into the peripheral blood. After a
further 20 hours they lose their RNA and become mature erythrocytes. Normally
the reticulocyte count does not exceed 2.0% of all red cells. The development from
proerythroblast to erythrocyte involves 3 or 4 cell divisions and takes 4 to 6 days.
About 1 in 8 or 1 in 16 erythroblasts fails to mature, and the cell is phagocytized
in the marrow. This can be detected biochemically by feeding labeled glycine when
excretion of labeled heme occurs in the feces within the first week. The major
excretion of labeled heme occurs at the end of the life-span of the red cells 110
days later. The term ineffective hemopoiesis refers to those cells dying in early
development.

Granulopoiesis

The earliest recognizable precursor is the myeloblast, which, in appearance, is not dissimilar to the proerythroblast. It lacks the perinuclear clear zone of the proerythroblast. After mitotic division granules appear in the cytoplasm, and the cell is termed a promyelocyte. Further maturation involves loss of nucleoli from the nucleus and the appearance of specific granules in the cytoplasm (neutrophil, eosinophil, and basophil). These cells are termed myelocytes. Early myelocytes still divide but later ones do not. Further maturation involves evolution of the nucleus into a horseshoe or band form and, finally, into the familiar lobular configuration of the polymorphonuclear leukocyte. The time from myeloblast to myelocyte is 7 to 8 days. Thereafter the band form or metamyelocyte remains in the marrow for a further 6 to 7 days before maturation into a polymorph. The half-time of the polymorph in the peripheral blood is only some 7 hours when it departs for the tissues. There may be 4 to 5 cell divisions between myeloblast to myelocyte. In normal marrow, granulocytic precursors outnumber normoblasts by 2- to 20-fold. More than half the granulocytes are at the metamyelocyte polymorph stage of development.

Megakaryocytes are seen as giant multinuclear cells under low power of the microscope. But giant cells with single large nucleus are also present and contain platelet demarcation membranes by which the cytoplasm is subdivided into future platelets. These platelets appear as strings from the edges of the cytoplasm.

In addition, normal marrow contains lymphocytes, macrophages, plasma cells, and, especially in marrow from children, osteoblasts. Marrows also show a very early cell that develops into a basophilic hemopoietic cell and is loosely termed a reticulum cell. It has a diffuse lacy cytoplasm with pink azurophil granules and a round nucleus with very distinctive round or oval nucleoli, which may take on a deep purple color in Romanowsky stains. They can be plentiful in actively erythropoietic marrows and presumably are the earliest recognizable red cell precursor. Cells can be seen in which the cytoplasm is in transition from a diffuse lacy pattern to deep basophilia. Their equivalent has not been described in *in vitro* cultures.

Lymphocyte Development

B Lymphocytes

The earliest development in B-cell maturation is a rearrangement of genetic material on chromosome 14 concerned with immunoglobulin synthesis. This is followed by the appearance in the cell cytoplasm of μ chains (the heavy chains of the immunoglobulin molecule). These cells are termed pre-B lymphocytes, and they give rise to small B lymphocytes, which now have IgM surface immunoglobulin. These represent the majority of B cells in marrow. The cells are ready to enter the peripheral blood (51).

T Lymphocytes

The early cells (? prothymocytes) develop in marrow. They become cells that acquire an enzyme terminal deoxynucleotidyltransferase (TdT) and in the mouse can be identified with an antiserum recognizing an antigen Thy-1. Further development of this cell occurs in the thymus gland. The majority of T cells in marrow, however, are circulating postthymic cells.

REQUIREMENTS FOR HEMOPOIESIS

In addition to the normal requirements of nutrients common to all cells, hemopoietic cells are particularly vulnerable to lack of iron, cobalamin (vitamin B_{12}), and folate. The bulk of iron in the body in man (some 2.5 g) is present in hemoglobin. The rapid turnover of hemopoietic cells makes them particularly vulnerable to lack of either folic acid or cobalamin. These are required for normal synthesis of purines and pyrimidines, which are the basic components of DNA and RNA. Their lack gives rise to an anemia wherein the red blood cells are abnormally larger (macrocytic) and the appearance of marrow cells becomes abnormal and is termed megaloblastic hemopoiesis. This is reversed by supplying either cobalamin or folate. Rarely a limiting factor to hemopoiesis in man may be lack of ascorbic acid, pyridoxine, or vitamin E.

ASSESSMENT OF MARROW ACTIVITY

A normal peripheral blood count implies normal marrow function. Marrow itself can be sampled by aspiration through a small needle inserted under local anesthetic into the marrow either in the region of the sterum or iliac crest. Marrow films are spread in the same way that peripheral blood films are made and cellularity and morphology assessed after fixation and staining. A core of marrow may be obtained under local anesthetic from the iliac crest and sectioned to show architecture as well as morphology of cells.

Distribution of hemopoietic marrow can be shown with short-lived iron isotopes (^{52}Fe), which will give a suitable picture using a gamma camera. Iron studies with longer lived iron isotopes (^{59}Fe) when given with plasma so that the iron is bound to transferrin show the sites of iron uptake (using surface counting) and the subsequent incorporation of that iron into red cells over the next 2 weeks. Normally such iron goes to marrow (maximum radioactive counts over the sacrum) and thereafter appears in the red cells. DNA synthesis can be studied with suspensions of marrow cells. For example, the conversion of deoxyuridine into thymidine and the incorporation of the latter into DNA can be assessed in a test called the deoxyuridine suppression test (26). Many other enzyme pathways can be studied using marrow cell preparations. A detailed account of the morphology of human marrow is provided in any standard text on hematology.

REFERENCES

1. Allen, T. D. (1981): Haemopoietic microenvironments in vitro: ultrastructural aspects. In: Microenvironments in Haemopoietic and Lymphoid Differentiation. *Ciba Foundation Symposium* 84, pp. 38–60. Pitman, London.

2. Bathija, A., Davis, S., and Trubowitz, S. (1979): Bone marrow adipose tissue: response to starvation. *Am. J. Hematol.*, 6:191–198.

3. Bentley, S. A. (1982): Bone marrow connective tissue and the haemopoietic microenvironment. *Br. J. Haematol.*, 50:1–6.

4. Bessis, M. (1958): L'ilot érythroblastique, unité fonctionelle de la moelle osseuse. *Rev. Hématol.*, 13:8–11.

5. Birgens, H. S., Ebbes, N. E., Karle, H., and Kristensen, L. Ø. (1983): Receptor binding of lactoferrin by human monocytes. *Br. J. Haematol.*, 54:383–391.

6. Broxmeyer, H. E., Smithyman, A., Eger, R. R., Meyers, P. A., and deSousa, M. (1978): Identification of lactoferrin as the granulocyte-derived inhibitor of colony-stimulating activity production. *J. Exp. Med.*, 148:1052–1067.

7. Castro-Malaspina, H., Gay, R. E., Resnick, G., Kapoor, N., Meyers, P., Chiarieri, D., McKenzie, S., Broixmeyer, H. E., and Moore, M. A. S. (1980): Characterization of human bone marrow fibroblast colony-forming cells (CFU/F) and their progeny. *Blood*, 56:289–301.

8. Chanarin, S., Barkhan, P. Peacock, M., and Stamp, T. C. B. (1964): Acute arrest of haemopoiesis. *Br. J. Haematol.*, 10:43–49.

9. Cline, M. J., and Fitchen, J. H. (1978): Inhibition of granulopoiesis. In: *Hemopoietic Cell Differentiation* (ICN-UCLA Symposia on Molecular and Cellular Biology, Vol. X) edited by D. W. Golde, M. J. Cline, D. Metcalf and C. E. Fox, pp. 461–469. Academic Press, New York.

10. Cotes, M. (1982): Immunoreactive erythropoietin in serum. I. Evidence for the validity of the assay method and the physiological relevance of estimates. *Br. J. Haematol.*, 50:427–438.

11. Dexter, T. M., and Moore, M. A. S. (1977): In vitro duplication and 'cure' of haemopoietic defects in genetically anaemic mice. *Nature (Lond.)*, 269:412–414.

12. Ebbe, S. (1979): Experimental and clinical megakaryocytopoiesis. *Clin. Haematol.* 8:371–394.

13. Fitchen, J. H. (1981): Granulocyte differentiation and culture. In: *Leucocyte Function*, edited by M. J. Cline, pp. 104–129. Churchill, Livingstone, New York.

14. Friedenstein, A. J., Chailakhyan, R. K., Latsinik, N. V., Pansyuk, A. F., and Keiliss-Borok, I. V. (1974): Stromal cells responsible for transferring the microenvironment of the hemopoietic tissues. *Transplantation*, 17:331–340.

15. Frisch, R. E., Canick, J. A., and Tulchinsky, D. (1980): Human fatty marrow aromatizes androgen to estrogen. *J. Clin. Endocrinol. Metab.* 51:394–396.

16. Greenberger, J. S. (1978): Sensitivity of corticosteroid-dependent, insulin-resistant lipogenesis in marrow preadipocytes of mutation diabetic-obese mice. *Nature*, 275:752–754.

17. Hann, I. M., Bodger, M. P., and Hoffbrand, A. V. (1983): Development of pluripotential hemopoietic progenitor cells in the human fetus. *Blood*, 62:118–123.

18. Hibbin, J. A., Njoku, O. S., Catovsky, D., and Goldman, J. M. (1983): Megakaryocyte progenitor cells (CFU-MK) in the blood of normal individuals and patients with myelofibrosis. *Exp. Hematol.*, (11 *Suppl*), 14:16.

19. Hudson, G., and Shortland, J. R. (1980): In: *The Reticuloendothelial System*, edited by I. Carr and W. T. Daems, pp. 329–360. Plenum Press, New York.

20. Knospe, W. H., Husseini, S. and Trobaugh, F. E. (1978): Hematopoiesis on cellulose ester membranes (CEM). II. Enrichment of the hematopoietic environment by the addition of selected cellular elements. *Exp. Hematol.*, 6:601–612.

21. Lasky, L. C., Ash, R. C., Kersey, J. H., Zanjani, E. D., and McCullough, J. (1982): Collection of pluripotential hematopoietic stem cells by cytaphoresis. *Blood*, 59:822–827.

22. Lichtman, M. A. (1981): The ultrastructure of the hemopoietic environment of the marrow: A review. *Exp. Hematol.*, 9:391–410.

23. Lipton, J. M., and Nathan, D. G. (1983): Cell-cell interactions in the regulation of erythropoiesis. *Br. J. Haematol.*, 53:361–367.

24. Messner, H. A., Fauser, A. A., Lepine, J., and Martin, M. (1980): Properties of human pluripotent hemopoietic progenitors. *Blood Cells*, 6:595–607.

25. Metcalf, D. (1979): Detection and analysis of human granulocyte-monocyte precursors using semisolid cultures. *Clin. Haematol.* 8:263–285.

26. Metz, J., Kelly, A., Swett, V. C., Waxman, S., and Herbert, V. (1968): Deranged DNA synthesis by bone marrow from vitamin B_{12}-deficient humans. *Br. J. Haematol.* 14:575–592.

27. Micklem, H. S. (1979): B lymphocytes, T lymphocytes and lymphopoiesis. *Clin. Haematol.* 8:395–419.
28. Monette, F. C., Holden, S. A., and Sheehy, M. J. (1983): The administration of hemin *in-vivo* augments the frequency and cycling of BFU-E but not CFU-E in murine bone marrow. *Exp. Hematol.*, [11, *Suppl.*] 14:26.
29. Moore, M. A. S. (1979): Humoral regulation of granulopoiesis. *Clin. Haematol.*, 8:287–309.
30. Myoshi, I., Irino, S., and Hiraki, K. (1966): Fibroblast-like transformation of human bone marrow fat cells in-vitro. *Exp. Cell Res.*, 41:220–223.
31. Nathan, D. G., Chess, L., Hillman, D. G., Clarke, B., Beard, J., Merler, E., and Houseman, D. E. (1978): Human erythroid burst-forming unit : T-cell requirement for proliferation *in-vivo*. *J. Exp. Med.*, 147:324–339.
32. Patt, H. M., and Maloney, M. A. (1970): Reconstitution of bone marrow in a depleted medullary cavity. In: *Haemopoietic Cellular Proliferation*, edited by F. Stohlman, pp. 56–66, Grune and Stratton, New York.
33. Petursson, S. R., Chervenick, P. A. and McDonald, T. P. (1983): Comparison of thrombopoietin and megakaryocyte colony stimulating activity *in-vitro*. *Exp. Haematol.* [11, *Suppl.*] 14:19.
34. Pike, B., and Robinson, W. A. (1970): Human bone marrow colony growth in agar gel. *J. Cell. Physiol.*, 76:77–84.
35. Prchal, J. F., Adamson, J. W., Steinmann, L., and Fialkow, P. J. (1976): Human erythroid colony formation in-vitro: evidence for clonal origin. *J. Cell. Physiol.* 89:489–492.
36. Reid, C. D. L., Baptista, L. C., and Chanarin, I. (1981): Erythroid colony growth in-vitro from human peripheral blood null cells: evidence for regulation by T-lymphocytes and monocytes. *Br. J. Haematol.*, 48:155–164.
37. Reid, C. D. L., Baptista, L. C., and Prouse, P. J. (1983): Response of BFU_E to monocyte, T cell and serum growth factors in normal and anaemic patients with rheumatoid arthritis (R.A.) *Exp. Haematol.*, [11, *Suppl.*] 14:30.
38. Reid, C. D. L., Baptista, L. C., Deacon, R., and Chanarin, I. (1981): Megaloblastic change is a feature of colonies derived from an early erythroid progenitor (BFU-E) stimulated by monocytes in culture. *Br. J. Haematol.*, 49:551–561.
39. Reimann, J., and Burger, H. (1979): In-vitro proliferation of haemopoietic cells in the presence of adherent cell layers. II: Differential effect of adherent cell layers from different organs. *Exp. Hematol.*, 7:52–58.
40. Rowley, S. D., and Stuart, R. K. (1983): 4-hydroperoxycyclophosphamide (4H-C) effects on human pluripotential stem cells (CFU-GEMM) in-vitro. *Exp. Hematol.*, [11, *Suppl.*] 14:11.
41. Schofield, R. (1979): The pluripotent stem cell. *Clin. Haematol.* 8:221–237.
42. Schraber, J. W., Bartlett, P. F., Clark-Lewis, I., and Boyd, A. W. (1981): Lymphoid differentiation in-vitro. In: Microenvironments in Haemopoietic and Lymphoid Differentiation, *Ciba Foundation Symposium* 84, pp. 130–160, Pitman, London.
43. Singer, J. W., Keeting, A., and Fialkow, P. J. (1983): Evidence suggesting a common progenitor for hematopoietic and marrow stromal cells. *Exp. Hematol.*, [11, *Suppl.*] 14:4.
44. Tavassoli, M. (1974): Differential response of bone marrow and extramedullary adipose cells to starvation. *Experientia*, 30:424–425.
45. Tavassoli, M. (1974): Marrow adipose cells. Ultrastructural and histochemical characterization. *Arch. Path.*, 94:189–192.
46. Tavassoli, M. (1977): Intravascular phagocytosis in the rabbit bone marrow: A possible fate of normal senescent red cells. *Br. J. Haematol.*, 36:323–326.
47. Tavassoli, M., and Crosby, W. H. (1968): Transplantation of marrow to extramedullary sites. *Science*, 161:54–56.
48. Testa, N. G. (1979): Erythroid progenitor cells: their relevance for the study of haematological disease. *Clin. Haematol.*, 8:311–333.
49. Till, J. E., and McCulloch, E. A. (1961): A direct measurement of the radiation sensitivity of normal mouse bone marrow cells. *Radiat. Res.*, 14:213–222.
50. Trubowitz, S., and Bathija, A. (1977): Cell size and palmitate-1-^{14}C turnover of rabbit marrow fat. *Blood*, 49:599–605.
51. Vogler, L. B. (1982): Bone marrow B cell development. *Clin. Haematol.* 11:509–529.
52. Weiss, L. (1976): The hematopoietic microenvironment of the bone marrow: An ultrastructural study of the stroma in rats. *Anat. Rec.*, 186:161–184.

53. Weiss, L. (1981): In: Microenvironments in Haemopoietic and Lymphoid Differentiation, *Ciba Foundation Symposium* 84, pp. 5–14, Pitman, London.
54. Zuckerman, K. S., Bagby, G., McCall, E., Patel, V., and Goodrum, D. (1983): Production of human erythroid burst promoting activity by human endothelial cells is stimulated by a monokine. *Exp. Hematol.*, [11, *Suppl.*] 14:40.

Toxicology of the Blood and Bone Marrow,
edited by Richard D. Irons. Raven Press,
New York © 1985.

Regulation and Structure of Hemopoiesis: Its Application in Toxicology

Eugene P. Cronkite

Medical Research Center, Brookhaven National Laboratory, Upton, New York 11973

STRUCTURE OF HEMOPOIESIS

There is an orderly flow of cells from the primitive self-renewing stem cell to early cytologically unidentifiable progenitors of erythrocytes, granulocytes, and platelets. These early progenitors expand exponentially and feed into the cytologically identifiable precursors of the three major hemopoietic cell lines (erythrocytic, granulocytic, and megakaryocytic) during which exponential expansion continues. This is shown schematically in Fig. 1. The regulation of self-renewal and commitment is not well understood. The age structure of the pluripotent stem cell pool is discussed later. The amplification process is discussed under erythropoiesis and granulopoiesis.

THE SELF-RENEWING STEM CELL POOL

The stem cell pool can be assayed quantitatively only in the mouse and rat. The assay method was developed by Till and McCulloch (84). A graded number of bone marrow cells (10^4–5×10^4) from a donor mouse are injected intravenously into a fatally irradiated mouse. Nodules, which can be counted under low-power magnification, form on the spleen surface from 7 to 14 days. The spleen colonies are clones (7). Self-renewal and differentiation into the three major cell lines take place in the spleen colonies (85). The cell that actually forms the spleen colony is called the colony-forming unit spleen (CFU-S), which is a fraction of the total colony-forming cell spleen (CFC-S). The fraction of CFC-S that actually settles in the spleen and produces spleen colonies varies from 0.05 to 0.2, depending on the strain of mouse and the time that one allows the spleen colonies to form.

There are problems with the assay. First, it is necessary to expose the assay mice to a fatal dose of radiation. Second, if one uses enough bone marrow cells to prevent death of the recipient mice, the number of colonies produced is large, becomes confluent, and cannot be counted. Thus, 5×10^3 to 6×10^4 bone marrow cells are used by most investigators. This number of bone marrow cells will not rescue the mice from the fatal dose of radiation necessary to prevent growth of endogenous colonies. Depending on the strain, age of mice, and the dose of

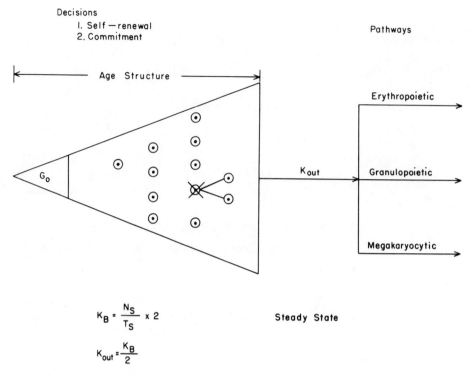

FIG. 1. Concept of the stem cell pool. K_B, birth rate; N_s, number of stem cells in DNA synthesis; T_s, average time for DNA synthesis; K_{out}, flux out of the stem cell pool by differentiation in "steady-state" hemopoiesis.

radiation used, mice may commence dying by the eighth day after irradiation, with very few, if any, surviving to the 14th day. Many investigators accordingly shortened the assay time to 9, 8, or 7 days. Seven days became popular because it was rare for mice to die; thus the assay was cheaper and more efficient.

In 1963 Siminovitch et al. (80) studied the abundance of self-renewing CFU-S in individual colonies 10, 12, and 14 days after marrow transplantation. CFU-S were present in colonies on days 10, 12, and 14, there being more per colony on day 14, with data based in some instances on a single surviving mouse. Till et al. in 1964 (85) extended these studies, finding that more than 50% of 10-day colonies contained CFU-S and that more than 90% of 12-day colonies contained CFU-S. From their data they concluded that two processes influence the CFU-S that lodge in the spleen. One is self-renewal and the other is differentiation to a non-self-renewing line (erythrocytic, granulocytic, megakaryocytic). If a stem cell lands in an area of spleen conducive to erythropoiesis, it may differentiate and thus the colony formed will not contain CFU-S. Alternatively, it may self-renew one or more times and the progeny, by chance, may differentiate into one or all of the three major lines, producing single or mixed colonies with or without CFU-S. The stochastic model states that $P_2 + P_0 = 1.0$, where P_2 = probability of self-renewal with a net gain of 1 CFU-S after mitosis, and P_0 = probability of differentiation.

Monte Carlo calculations were made with $P_2 = 0.6$ and $P_0 = 0.4$ to determine how many colonies would contain N or fewer CFU-S, where N equals the number of CFU-S per colony. There was a very good correlation between observed data and the stochastic model. Progeny of single CFU-S behave randomly in respect to self-renewal and/or differentiation, whereas the population of hemopoietic cells at large in the intact animal has an orderly behavior that regulates the whole by changing the self-renewal and differentiation probabilities up or down as needed. Vogel et al. in 1968 (86) found that the self-renewal probabilities of CFU-S in spleen colonies during growth between 8 to 13 days were 0.62, providing expansion of the CFU-S pool. Nakahata et al. (65) extended studies on the stochastic nature of self-renewal with results comparable to Till et al. (85) and Vogel et al. (86).

That one can affect the differentiation of stem cells and amplification into colonies has been established. Liron and Feldman in 1965 (56) showed that trans-fusion plethora nearly abolished the formation of erythroid colonies from CFU-S whereas granulocytic colonies increased to some extent. This effect was reversed by erythropoietin (8). These studies were performed on 11-day spleen colonies. The content of CFU-S in the colonies was not measured. Preisler and Henderson (71), however, showed that the total CFU-S content of bone marrow and spleen is increased by plethora. Schofield and Lajtha (78) showed that the total CFU-S content of the spleen increased exponentially from day 6 to day 15 after injection of 3×10^4 bone marrow cells. When larger numbers of bone marrow cells are injected, the exponential growth declines after 10 days, indicating that P_2 is approaching 0.5 or a "steady-state" production of stem cells. Their studies also indicate that the time between transplantation and onset of CFU-S proliferation is inversely related to the number of bone marrow cells injected.

Studies by Rosendaal et al. (76) and Hellman et al. (46) resulted in the notion that stem cells are organized on the basis of their generation age. Hodgson and Bradley (48) introduced the term "pre-CFU-S." This is a primitive stem cell in a G_0 state since it survives treatment with fluorouracil (5-FU) and other agents that kill cells in DNA synthesis. Patt et al. (67) and Hagan and MacVittie (41) perfused mice with bromodeoxyuridine (BrdUrd), which is incorporated into DNA, sensi-tizing the cells to ultraviolet light (254 nm). When cell suspensions of the bone marrow of such treated mice were exposed to UV light after different infusion times of BrdUrd, the kill of the CFU-S increased exponentially with BrdUrd infusion time. It was concluded that less than 10% of the CFU-S are in a prolonged G_0-G_1 and that most of the CFU-S population have a relatively short proliferative history, thus giving an estimate of the size of the "pre-CFU-S" pool of cells.

Salner et al. (77) showed that the CFU-S population could be separated by peanut agglutinin lectin into high and low self-renewal fractions. Botnick et al. (9) extended these studies to show that the stem cell compartment is a continuum of cells whose self-renewal capacity varies inversely with their mitotic history. Thus, it has been known since the early 1960s that the CFU-S are most prevalent in the

11- to 14-day colonies, and over the last 10 years it has been shown that the hemopoietic stem cell pool has an age structure based on its past proliferative history. Recent studies (45,57) have rekindled interest in spleen colony formation and the nature of the cells that produce colonies in the spleen at different time intervals after transplantation of bone marrow cells. These recent publications make seminal contributions on the properties of cells that produce colonies visible at 7 to 9 or 14 days. For example, Magli et al. (57) investigated the significance of the spleen colony assay. They exteriorized and photographed the spleen on day 8 and again on day 10. Some colonies seen on day 8 had disappeared and others not visible on day 8 had appeared by day 10. Their results imply that the spleen colony assay provides a measure of pluripotential stem cells capable of extensive proliferation, only when macroscopic colonies are scored at 11 days or later. Their observations are of interest, but do not conclusively demonstrate that the early 7- to 8-day colonies are not derived from CFU-S with a limited self-renewal capacity if one accepts the stochastic model of stem cell self-renewal and differentiation elaborated by Till et al. (85), Vogel et al. (86), and Nakahata et al. (65). Some of the early colonies will have been derived from CFU-S and others may have been derived from early erythrocytic progenitors. Resolution of the problem by experiment will be intricate. In fact, there is no appropriate control to show that exteriorization of the spleen did not cause the colonies to disappear.

All cells in the course of progressive differentiation develop an increasing number and diversity of surface receptors for molecules that influence their metabolic and synthetic functions, rates of proliferation, etc. For example, CFU-S and early burst-forming unit erythroid (BFU-E) do not have receptors for erythropoietin whereas late BFU-E and CFU-E have increasing numbers of receptors for erythropoietin. As cells progressively differentiate, surface antigenic characteristics change. Harris et al. (45) clearly showed that there is a distinct antigenic difference between murine stem cells that produce 8-day colonies as compared with stem cells that produce 14-day colonies. The 14-day colony corresponds to the pre-CFU-S (48).

In addition to the heterogeneity in respect to mitotic reserve and surface receptors of the pluripotent stem cell pool, discussed above, other heterogeneities are known. Monette and DeMellow (64) demonstrated that more stem cells in G_0-G_1 seed the spleen than CFU-S in DNA synthesis. Inoue et al. (49) showed that CFU-S in DNA synthesis have a preference for seeding in the bone marrow. Inoue and Cronkite (50) showed that the number of 7-day colony formers increases with the age of the mice from 1.12×10^3 per femur at 42 days of age to 4.34×10^3 at 763 days of age. At the same time the size of the colonies produced by the aged CFU-S is much smaller. The increase in the number of CFU-S with decreased colony size is compatible with diminution in number of pre-CFU-S and the production of more CFU-S with lower self-renewal capacity. In 1984 Chertkov and Drize (20) pursued further the case of the disappearing colonies and showed that the precursors of the transient spleen colonies proliferate more rapidly than the precursors forming 11-day colonies.

In vitro techniques for the assay of a pluripotent stem cell have been developed for man (30,31,60,61) and mouse (42). In the mouse the *in vitro* pluripotent stem cell (CFU-mix) responds to erythropoietic stimulation and suppression as does the CFU-S, suggesting that they may be identical cells. The possibility that the CFU-mix is a pluripotent cell without or little self-renewal capacity remains.

In summary, observations on the self-renewal and commitment of the hemopoietic stem cells during the last 23 years are as follows:

1. A hierarchy of multipotential hemopoietic stem cells assayable *in vivo*, and to a lesser extent *in vitro*, exists. The earliest stem cells ("pre-CFU-S") have a very high self-renewal capacity and are clearly of most importance in establishing a successful bone marrow transplant, but are not necessarily the sole target cell for leukemogenesis.

2. Self-renewal and commitment to differentiation of the primitive hemopoietic stem cells are controlled by a stochastic process. The probability for self-renewal (*p*) is regulated by demand for replenishment of stem cells (regeneration $p > 0.5$) or more differentiated progeny (erythrocytes after bleeding or in hypoxia and granulocytes in infection). Thus it is probable that *p* is either directly or indirectly controlled by humoral molecular factors produced within or without the bone marrow.

3. There is a continuum from the most immature stem cell with extensive self-renewal capacity through pluripotent-committed stem cells (producers of mixed colonies of all cell types—RBC, granulocytes, macrophage, and megakaryocytes), tri- or bipotent progenitors, and monopotent progenitors (one cell type in the colony).

4. The homing of injected CFU-S differs, depending on whether they are in G_0-G_1 or S.

5. The *in vitro* culture of a cell that produces mixed colonies (erythrocytic, megakaryocytic, macrophagic, and granulocytic) suggests that it may be identical to the self-renewing CFU-S.

TRANSIT CELL POPULATIONS—AMPLIFICATION OF STEM CELL INPUT

The well-characterized transit populations are the erythrocytic and granulocytic-monocytic. These in turn are divided into the cytologically unidentifiable and identifiable populations. There are two ways in which the production rate can be increased: (a) an increased stem cell input and (b) an increased amplification by more cell divisions of the stem cell input. For every additional mitosis in the transit population, the output is doubled. Figure 2 portrays erythropoiesis schematically and Fig. 3, granulopoiesis.

With the development of techniques for the assay of early, apparent non-self-renewing progenitors of differentiated cell lines, spleen colonies were assayed for their presence. The early progenitors are granulocyte-monocyte colony-forming unit in culture (GM-CFU-C), 3- and 8-day BFU-E, and colony-forming unit eryth-

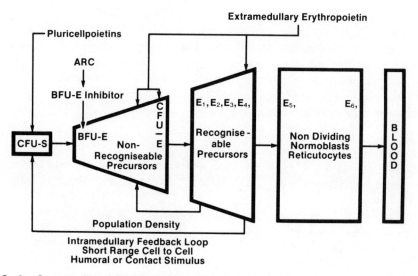

FIG. 2. Concept of intramedullary regulation of the rate of red cell production. ARC, adventitial reticular cell; CFU-S, BFU-E, and CFU-E are defined in text; E_1-E_4, the cytologically identifiable mitotable erythrocytic precursors; E_5, reticulocyte; E_6, mature red cell.

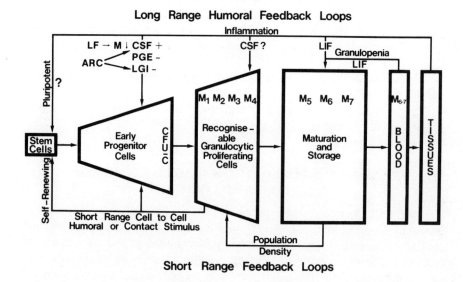

FIG. 3. Concept of regulation of the rate of production of granulocytes. LF, lactoferrin; M, monocyte-macrophage; CSF, colony-stimulating factor; PGE, prostaglandin; ARC, adventitial reticular cell; LIF, leukocytosis-inducing factor; M_1–M_4, myeloblast through myelocyte; M_5, metamyelocyte; M_6, band neutrophil; M_7, segmented neutrophil.

roid (CFU-E). Gregory and Henkelman (40) determined the fraction of 11- to 12-day spleen colonies that contained varying numbers of each progenitor. The CFU-S were not detected in 67.5% of the spleen colonies, and CFU-S content varied from one to several hundred per colony. Failure to detect a CFU-S in a colony does not imply that the colony was not derived from a CFU-S because of the stochastic nature of a CFU-S being induced to self-renew or to differentiate as described earlier. The possibility that a visible colony was derived from an early progenitor such as BFU-E or GM-CFU-C remains, since these precursors can, at least *in vitro*, produce colonies of 50,000 cells (46). Pure erythrocytic colonies as large as 10^7 cells have been observed in 7-day spleen colonies by Reincke et al. (74). This requires a minimum of 24 consecutive doubling divisions. It is unlikely that a cell in a terminal pathway will have that large a mitotic reserve, implying that colonies of that size probably arose from a pluripotent stem cell.

STRUCTURE OF THE ERYTHROCYTIC TRANSIT POPULATION

By *in vitro* culture methods it has been shown that there is a continuum of cells increasing in number by mitosis. This cytologically unidentifiable population has been divided into BFU-E and CFU-E. The BFU-E is a cell that produces colonies greater than 64 cells or multiple grape-like clusters of cells. The CFU-E is a cell that produces a colony of 8 to 64 cells. The BFU-E- and CFU-E-derived colonies are identified by staining with benzidine, demonstrating presence of hemoglobin (2,3,40,82). In turn, for practical reasons in the mouse, the BFU-E are divided into 8- and 3-day categories, the 8-day BFU-E being closest to the pluripotent stem cell and the 3-day BFU-E being intermediate between the 8-day BFU-E and the 2-day CFU-E. These entities are enumerated by the size, shape of the colonies produced, and their dependence on erythropoietin and other factors. They can be grown in methylcellulose or plasma clots. The 3- to 8-day BFU-E requires a relatively high concentration of erythropoietin, 2.5 units per ml of culture along with an ill-defined burst-promoting activity. CFU-E requires only 0.25 unit of erythropoietin per ml of culture. Stephenson et al. (82) and Axelrad et al. (2,3) published the details for culture of CFU-E and BFU-E for mouse and man. Recently, the CFU-E have been shown to have a time-dependence on the presence of erythropoietin (69).

The CFU-E feed into the cytologically identifiable erythrocytic precursors (proerythroblast, basophilic erythroblast, polychromatophilic, and orthochromatic normoblasts). Exponential growth continues through the polychromatophilic stage. The identifiable erythrocytic precursors and the CFU-E compartment are responsive to demand control. Hypertransfusion of red cells drastically reduces the number of identifiable erythrocytic precursors and the CFU-E. There is little change in the BFU-E. Anemia induced by bleeding or hemolysis increases the number of CFU-E, with relatively little change in the BFU-E compartments (43). The acceleration of erythropoiesis by hypoxia and erythropoietin has been reviewed in detail by Miller et al. (63).

The regulation of erythropoiesis is shown schematically in Fig. 2. It is generally believed that erythropoietin is the major molecule that regulates the rate of red cell production. Erythropoietin is produced in the kidney. Hypoxia, hemolysis, and/or bleeding result in a prompt increase in serum erythropoietin concentration accelerating production at the CFU-E and in the recognizable erythropoietic precursors, increasing the number of mitoses, shortening the transit time, and increasing the rate of hemoglobin synthesis. It is to be noted that erythropoietin probably is not the sole regulator of erythropoiesis. Plethora inhibits proliferation of recognizable erythrocytic precursors and CFU-E allowing BFU-E to remain relatively constant with a small increase in the size of the CFU-S pool. Reincke et al. (73) showed that depletion of the recognizable erythrocytic pool by radio iron erythrocytocide results in a prompt diminution of the CFU-S pool, implying an intramedullary feedback loop that induces rapid differentiation of CFU-S into the erythrocytic pathway in the absence of changes in concentration of erythropoietin in serum or changes in the red cell mass. In addition, Cronkite et al. (25) produced evidence that a culture of the adventitial reticular cell derived from bone marrow produces an inhibitor of BFU-E proliferation. It is seen that erythropoiesis is regulated by a complex series of positive and negative feedback loops. Hypoxia, hemolysis, and bleeding stimulate a positive feedback loop by increasing erythropoietin concentration in the serum. Plethora institutes a negative feedback loop suppressing erythropoiesis. In addition, an intramedullary loop based on population density of the recognizable erythrocytic precursors induces a forced differentiation of CFU-S into the erythrocytic pathway when it is reduced in size (73).

THE RED CELL

The orthochromatic normoblast extrudes its nucleus, becoming a reticulocyte that continues to synthesize hemoglobin until its supply of mRNA is exhausted, at which time it is a mature red cell in man with a normal average life-span of 120 days. It is of interest to note that Winifred Ashby (1) in 1919 determined the life-span of the human red cell to be 120 days by differential agglutination of transfused red cells. Approximately 20 to 30 years later her work was confirmed utilizing the stable N-15-glycine labeling of heme by Shemin and Rittenberg (79) and with chromium-51 labeling by Gray and Sterling (39). The red cell life-span allows calculation of red cell death rates which, for example, in human beings are 0.83% per day. Shorter life-spans will result in greater daily turnover of red cells. Human beings are able to compensate for increased destruction of red cells up to approximately six times the normal production rate.

The most practical method today of measuring red cell life-span is by labeling the subject cells with chromium-15 potassium dichromate, washing the cells, giving an autotransfusion, and measuring the rate of disappearance of the labeled cells. This technique is applicable in all mammals.

Iron uptake in the peripheral RBCs has been used as an index of injury to erythropoietic precursors and pluripotent stem cells (55). This approach is based, in part, on the assumption that iron is incorporated only into the erythrocytic precursors from the proerythroblast through the reticulocyte where heme and hemoglobin are being synthesized. This assumption is not true. All cells synthesize some iron-containing enzymes such as cytochrome. The amount of ^{59}Fe incorporated into hemoglobin or heme synthesizing cells is much greater than in other cells. In fact, radio ^{59}Fe has been used to measure granulocytic life-span by Resegotti (75). Although it is true that at 24 hours or longer a suppressed uptake of radio ^{59}Fe indicates injury to erythropoiesis, it is difficult to pinpoint with accuracy the level in the erythropoietic pathway at which the injury has occurred. It is better to use a direct assay of the CFU-S, 3-8-day BFU-E, CFU-E, and to count quantitatively the identifiable erythrocytic precursors in the bone marrow.

GRANULOCYTIC-MONOCYTE TRANSIT POPULATION

Granulopoiesis is shown schematically in Fig. 3. Independently, Pluznik and Sachs (70) and Bradley and Metcalf (10) cloned precursors of granulocytes and macrophages in a semisolid agar culture. The colonies are granulocytic, macrophagic, or mixed granulocytic-macrophagic colonies. The precursor is called the granulocyte-macrophage colony-forming unit in culture (GM-CFU-C). GM colony formation requires the continual presence of specific colony-stimulating molecules (CSF). If these molecules are removed, growth ceases. The molecules are alpha-1 glycoproteins of 45,000 to 60,000 daltons. One unit of CSF is that amount that produces one colony. CSF has been purified so that 1 mg contains 1.6×10^8 units by Stanley et al. (81). Later studies identified and isolated molecular entities that primarily stimulate the GM-CFU-C to form macrophagic, granulocytic, or mixed granulocyte-macrophage colonies. If one initiates a culture with macrophage colony-stimulating factor (M-CSF) for 3 to 5 mitoses and then washes out M-CSF, reclones, and adds granulocyte-macrophage colony-stimulating factor (GM-CSF), predominately macrophage colonies are formed. The initiation of a culture with GM-CSF followed by recloning M-CSF results in GM or G colonies. The bipotential GM-CFU-C are, after 3 to 5 mitoses, irreversibly committed by M-CSF to produce macrophage colonies and by GM-CSF to produce GM, G, or M colonies (62). Thus, M-CSF suppresses gene(s) responsible for differentiation of GM-CFU-C into granulocytes and GM-CSF suppresses gene(s) responsible for differentiation into pure macrophage colonies.

In soft agar, culture colonies are defined as an aggregate containing 50 or more cells. Fewer cells are defined as a cluster. If one counts the number of cells in the aggregates, one finds that the largest colonies are the fewest in number and the smaller clusters largest in number. It would appear then that there should be an exponentially increasing number of progenitors that produce colonies of decreasing size. If in the continuum of cells from the CFU-S through the GM-CFU-C to the terminal myelocyte mitosis an additional mitosis is added to some proliferating clones, the output will increase. If all clones are induced to have an additional mitosis, the output will double (26).

TABLE 1. *Cellular and mitotic characteristics of the granulopoietic pathway*

Cellular pool	Granulopoiesis	Characteristics	Mitotic capacity
PSC	Stem cell	Self-renewing and responsive to differentiation	Extensive—possibly greater than 100 mitoses
Bipotent stem cell unidentifiable	GM-CFU-C	Responsive to M-CSF or GM-CSF Amplifies stem cell input	Up to 20 mitoses
Identifiable multiplicative	Myeloblast Promyelocyte Myelocyte	Further amplification and maturation	About 4–5 mitoses
Maturation	Metamyelocyte Band neutrophil Segmented	Maturation—development of functional enzymes, mobility, and phagocytosis	None
Functional	Segmented blood neutrophil	Function—fight infection Responsive to chemotaxis	None
Cell death	Random loss and pyknosis	Random or senescent death	

The number of colonies observed in an *in vitro* culture of GM-CFC is dependent on the concentration of CSF in the culture. The number increases from zero to a maximum in a sigmoid manner reaching a plateau. The concentration of CSF on the plateau is used for assays for the abundance of GM-CFU-C in bone marrow or blood. At the plateau level of CSF the number of colonies is proportionate to the number of bone marrow cells plated. The cells producing clusters feed into the cytologically identifiable granulocytic precursors—myeloblast, promyelocyte, myelocyte, metamyelocyte, band neutrophil, and segmented marrow granulocytes. The kinetics of the identifiable granulocytic precursors have been well established and reviewed by Cronkite and Vincent (26).

Tritiated thymidine (^{3}HTdR) has been used to "flash" label cells in DNA synthesis and observe their subsequent behavior (dilution of label and flow from a proliferative compartment to nondividing maturation compartments and entrance into the bloodstream). DNA synthesis time in human granulocytic and erythrocytic lines has been shown to be 11 to 14 hours (83). In Table 1 the structure and properties of granulocytic precursors are shown. The kinetics of human granulopoiesis are summarized from studies of Cronkite et al. (21,23–26) and Fliedner et al. (33,34):

1. The flux of precursors into the myeloblast is approximately 0.4×10^7/kg/hr.
2. There is one myeloblast mitosis after an average of 16 hours.
3. There is one promyelocytic mitosis after an average of 20 hours.
4. There are two successive myelocytic cycles of approximately 54 hours each.

5. A minimum of 3 hours' maturation is required for a myelocyte after terminal mitosis to become a metamyelocyte.
6. Metamyelocytes are replaced at a rate of approximately 3.3% per hour—turnover 30.3 hours.
7. The average turnover time of band cells is 49.9 hours.
8. The average turnover time of marrow granulocytes is 71.8 hours.
9. The emergence time from labeling to first appearance in the peripheral blood is 90 to 100 hours in normal hemopoiesis and has been reduced to 48 hours in bacterial infection.
10. The flow of labeled cells from myelocyte to the blood follows "first in–first out" pipeline kinetics (58).

PERIPHERAL BLOOD GRANULOCYTE

The life-span of granulocytes in the peripheral blood was largely a matter of conjecture until ^{32}P diisopropyl fluorophosphate (DFP 32) was introduced into the study of blood granulocytes by Professor Wintrobe's Salt Lake City group, reviewed by Cartwright et al. (19). Granulocytes enter the blood from the bone marrow, following which there is a random loss of the radioactively labeled cells. This exponential decrease is characterized by the granulocyte half-disappearance time $(T_{1/2})$. The average granulocyte life time is $T_{1/2}$ divided by ln 2 (0.693). The Salt Lake City group observed that about one-half the total neutrophils in the blood were circulating at one time, the others being marginated along the walls of venules and perhaps in the spleen. Kinetically, the total blood granulocyte pool (TBGP) behaves as a single entity, and the granulocyte turnover rate (GTR) equals $TBGP \times 0.693/T_{1/2}$. The studies of Dresch et al. (29) and Dancey et al. (27) utilizing other granulocyte-labeling techniques show that DFP 32 underestimates the half-time of granulocytes in the blood of man. Although DFP 32 underestimates the mean life-span of the granulocyte in the peripheral blood because of isotope elution *in vivo*, it does not alter the principles of granulocyte behavior in the blood. Granulocyte studies in the dog comparable to those reported above in man are published (28,58,59,66,67). None of the labeling techniques such as DFP 32, chromium 51, or tritiated thymidine is particularly useful for the usual toxicological studies. The *in vivo* labeling in mice or dogs with ^{125}I-deoxyuridine, a thymidine analog, labels granulocytes when the precursors are in DNA synthesis. At a later time, labeled granulocytes emerge into the peripheral blood, the time depending on the species, and then transfusions of these cells can be made into other recipients to determine the life-span.

Underlying the demonstration of a relatively short life-span for granulocytes in the peripheral blood with random loss of the labeled cells emerged the notion that all cells are migrating randomly into the tissues. A systematic study by Jamuar and Cronkite (51) in pathogen-free mice failed to detect any extravascular granulocytes even when animals had granulocyte counts of 300,000/mm³. The conclusion from this study was that granulocytes are removed selectively by the spleen and disintegrate in the bloodstream.

A few comments on the responsiveness of the granulocytic system are in order. Granulocytes have a major and perhaps sole function of searching for, phagocytizing, and killing bacteria to contain an infectious process. In the normal "steady state" in man, 3.5×10^7/kg/hr are produced and killed to maintain a constant pool of granulocytes ready to attack bacterial invaders. Infection requires enormous numbers of granulocytes in a short time in restricted volumes of tissue to erect a defensive wall and contain the bacterial invaders. At least three factors are critical. First, chemotactic mechanisms by which the organism directs a steady stream of granulocytes from the blood into and around the infected tissue. Second, demand control that mobilizes stores of granulocytes and increases the production rate. Third, intact phagocytic and bacterial killing mechanisms are essential.

Earlier, the bipotent precursor for granulocytes and monocyte macrophages was discussed. Human cyclic neutropenia shows us that granulocyte and monocyte production is closely linked. As the granulocytes tumble down there is a reciprocal increase in the monocytes. The ratio of monocyte to granulocyte turnover rates is 0.14. In the steady state seven granulocytes enter the blood for every monocyte. If one assumes that there is a steady production of GM-CFU-C, each of which can be fixed in its direction of differentiation by exposure to GM-CSF or M-CSF, then one is led to believe that intramedullary production of GM-CSF and M-CSF cycles so that more GM-CSF-C are directed into granulocyte production or that there is a smaller amplification of GM-CFU-C that are committed by M-CSF.

Granulocyte production rate is very responsive to sterile or bacterial inflammation. The first response is due to chemotaxis, which attracts huge numbers of granulocytes into the involved volume of tissue. This results in a fleeting granulopenia and simultaneous release or production of leukocytosis-inducing factor (38). The stored granulocytes in the bone marrow are rapidly released, resulting in a granulocytosis. The emergence time from the myelocyte to the blood is drastically reduced. For example, Cronkite et al. (23) showed in dogs submitted to sterile inflammation that the normal emergence time of approximately 60 hours decreases to 8 to 16 hours when inflammation has been induced 24 hours earlier. At the same time, the ratio of myelocytic to erythrocytic mitoses increases by a factor of three, and the fraction of myelocytes in DNA synthesis increases by a factor of approximately two. All of these observations point to an increased amplification at the terminal end of granulopoiesis. This does not preclude an increased input from the pluripotent stem cell pool. It does demonstrate that *in vivo* regulation does act, at least in part, by increasing amplification and decreasing transit time through the marrow. Such was suggested by *in vitro* studies of Metcalf (62), who showed that CSF accelerated maturation of granulocytes through increased RNA and protein synthesis along with enhancement of phagocytosis.

The molecular modulation of granulopoiesis has been investigated in detail by many (4–6,12–18,47,53,68). Broxmeyer et al. (12–17) demonstrated *in vitro* that prostaglandin partially inhibits the production of macrophage colonies by raising the threshold for CSF. Iron-saturated lactoferrin partially inhibits production of GM and M-CSF by monocytes and macrophages. Lactoferrin acts only on I_A

antigen-positive monocytes. The positive feedback loop is the production of GM or M-CSF increasing the production of granulocytes and/or monocytes. Prostaglandin (PGE) raises the threshold of the target cells for CSF and lactoferrin, and acidic isoferritins suppress the production of CSF, providing a negative feedback loop. Bagby et al. (5) demonstrated that monocytes in culture produce a monokine that stimulates a variety of cells (endothelial, fibroblasts, and T cells) to produce CSF. Bagby thus assigns a pivotal role to monocytes in regulating granulopoiesis. In addition to the roles assigned to macrophage production of CSF and PGE and partial inhibition of CSF by lactoferrin, other marrow cells are involved.

Bone marrow stromal cells were originally believed to be supporting cells. It has now been shown that a series of bone marrow cells will in culture produce molecular species that influence the rate of production of granulocytes. For example, in 1981 Harigaya et al. (44) were the first to isolate and clone a stromal cell from murine long-term bone marrow cultures that produce CSF. In 1982 Lanotte et al. (54) confirmed the production of CSF by another stromal cell line. In addition, Quesenberry and Gimbrone (72) isolated a human endothelial cell line (not from bone marrow) that also produced CSF. Furthermore, T lymphocytes under stimulation by lectins will produce CSF (4,6,47). The cell line isolated by Harigaya et al. (44) was characterized by Garnett et al. (35–37) and Cronkite et al. (25). This cell line, called H-1, was isolated from a long-term bone marrow culture and is most likely derived from an adventitial reticular cell; it produces CSF and a labile inhibitor of granulopoiesis.

In summary, *in vivo* and *in vitro* studies in man and animals tell us that granulopoiesis is responsive (Fig. 3). Upon peripheral demand there is usually a fleeting initial neutropenia as the blood granulocytes charge into the infected volume of tissue to set up a defensive perimeter against the bacteria. Neutropenia is followed by an increase in serum leukocytosis-inducing factor. This factor mobilizes the granulocyte reserves, which then stream into the blood producing a granulocytosis and reinforcing the initial defensive zone. As the marrow granulocytes are diminished in number, myelocytic mitoses increase in number, and the transit time from the myelocyte to emergence in the blood is reduced by a factor of three to four. GM-CFC increase in number and the entire mitotable pool expands. It is reasonable to ascribe these effects to an increased concentration of CSF within the marrow. Burlington et al. (18) believe that the intramedullary-increased production of CSF is stimulated by an as yet unidentified molecular species circulating from the periphery to the marrow. Alternatively, the simple reduction in size of the granulocyte population within the marrow may reduce the concentration of lactoferrin derived from intramedullary granulocytes allowing the marrow to accelerate production of granulocytes.

The production of factors that regulate differentiation, rates of proliferation, and maturation *in vitro* is a clear demonstration that genes for these regulatory proteins are in the genetic repertoire. It is reasonable to expect these regulatory proteins active *in vitro* to have an *in vivo* function. The paramount questions are:

1. Where are they produced?

2. How are the levels modulated up and down to change rates of production and to fulfill the momentary needs of the host *in vivo*?

For the adventitial reticular cell and/or other stromal cells to play an *in vivo* role in granulopoiesis as suggested, there must be programmed signals to genes in these cells to increase or decrease production of the stimulatory and inhibitory factors for granulopoiesis in order to meet the needs of the organism. These chemical signals are not identified. Recently, Kohsaki et al. (52) identified a factor from human urine that produces a granulocytosis but apparently does not have CSA activity and does not contain endotoxin. This may be the factor that we postulate, acting through stimulation of CSF production within the marrow.

What can one expect in the future? The structure of granulopoiesis is reasonably well known. The rates of movement from one part of the granulopoietic pathway to another are established. We need to know more about the regulation of these rates *in vivo*. Are there specific molecules arising from outside the marrow that home on specific receptors on cells of different levels of granulopoietic maturity in the marrow that are responsible for adjusting production rates to meet the needs of the organism? Is there a single peripheral chemical mediator that adjusts the release rate of granulocytes from the marrow? Will a decrease in the mature neutrophil population be adequate to trigger intramedullary production and release of humoral stimulators and inhibitors from stromal cells and to adjust the production rate up or down? Does the peripheral molecular signal act on the stromal cells, which in turn provide stimulatory and inhibitory molecules as needed?

OTHER HEMOPOIETIC CELL LINES

Space does not permit a detailed description of lymphopoiesis or thrombopoiesis. Both have structures analogous to erythropoiesis and granulopoiesis and are regulated by a series of stimulatory and inhibitory molecular feedback loops. When thrombopoiesis fails or is severely compromised resulting in platelet counts less than 50,000 per μl^3, the individual is in danger of spontaneous hemorrhage or inability to quench bleeding after minor trauma. When lymphopoiesis fails, an acquired immunodeficiency develops the characteristics that depend on whether B, T, or all lymphocytes are involved.

THE EFFECT OF TOXIC AGENTS ON HEMOPOIESIS

Figure 1 shows that reduction in number and differentiation of pluripotent stem cells (PSCs) will result in impaired production of red cells, granulocytes, and platelets unless there are compensatory mechanisms. Normally, a small fraction of PSCs are in cycle ($< 10\%$). As the PSC population diminishes in size, the fraction in DNA synthesis tends to increase, thus maintaining a relatively constant number in DNA synthesis.

The birth rate (K_B) is

$$K_B = \frac{N_s \times 2}{T_s}$$

where N_s = number in DNA synthesis and T_s = time for DNA synthesis. In a "steady state" $K_{out} = K_B/2$. Half of the progeny produced remain to replicate again and half differentiate. The critical decisions for the PSC are self-renewal or commitment, and little is known about the factors that regulate each.

Toxic agents may kill PSC in proportion to the dose of the agent. If the PSC is reduced below approximately 10% of its normal size, compensation as discussed above fails, and red cell, granulocyte, and platelet deficiencies develop (pancytopenia) at rates proportionate to the life-spans of the formed elements in the blood. In man granulopenia develops within a few days, thrombopenia within 2 to 4 weeks, and anemia when all red cell formation ceases at 0.83% per day.

Some agents may act as mutagens, altering or deleting certain genes so that the PSC may lose the capacity, in part or in whole, for differentiation into one or more of the cell lines, resulting in some degree of anemia, thrombopenia, or granulocytopenia. PSCs may also be genetically altered so that their progeny when directed down different pathways may produce mature cells with defective or absent enzymes or impaired membranes or motility. If the genetic injury to the PSC is not lethal and becomes fixed by mitosis into a viable but defective clone of PSC, defective progeny will be produced until the clone dies out by differentiation into a terminal transit population.

Erythropoiesis can, in general, be regulated up or down by altering the flow of PSC into erythropoiesis or by changing amplification of the transit population (Fig. 2). *Polycythemia vera* is a PSC disease. If the kidneys fail to produce erythropoietin in amounts sufficient to produce adequate stimulation of CFU-E and the recognizable erythrocytic precursors, an anemia will develop. This happens in chronic renal failure produced by renal toxins, genetic, autoimmune, or bacterial disease of the kidneys.

Some agents may act primarily on the transit population, blocking proliferation at any stage from BFU-E through the last dividing erythrocytic precursor. These agents may act through alkylating proteins, mRNA or DNA of the transit population. If the PSC is spared or has effective repair mechanisms, the injury to the transit population will disappear as the defective transit cells die out and are replaced from the PSC pool. Thus injury solely to a transit population is evanescent.

Some agents may act only on the mature red cell, shortening its life-span and producing a severe hemolytic anemia. Such an agent is phenyl hydrazine. Remove the agent and as the defective red cells are removed, they will be replaced by red cells of normal life-span at an accelerated rate. It is of interest that human beings can increase red cell production by at least a factor of six to compensate for chronic hemolysis.

If an animal or man is exposed to a toxic agent and an anemia develops, the following analysis may be done. Observe the morphology of the red cell. The presence of Heinz bodies suggests hemolysis. The presence of nuclear fragments (micronuclei) suggests damage to the transit erythroblasts. If micronuclei were to persist for long intervals after removal of the toxins, it would imply cytogenetic damage to PSC. If the red cell life-span is shortened, hemolysis is proved. If the red cell life-span is normal and anemia persists, red cell production is decreased. An examination of the bone marrow is helpful. A reduced myeloid erythroid ratio suggests a shrinkage of the recognizable erythrocytic precursors. If accompanied by a reduction in the number of CFU-E and BFU-E there is either a reduced influx of PSC into erythropoiesis or a reduced amplification of the total erythrocytic transit population. If there is a normal number of BFU-E and CFU-E with a reduced number of recognizable erythrocytic precursors, there is a block in the transit from the CFU-E to the erythroblast.

In the mouse one can also measure the PSC by the spleen colony assay for CFU-S. If CFU-S is reduced in size and has not compensated by increasing the fraction of CFU-S in DNA synthesis, there will be a diminished production of the three major cell lines. When PSC production is compromised there may be competition for a reduced number of PSC. In the presence of infection the production of granulocytes may go up at the expense of erythropoiesis, or in the presence of hypoxia erythropoiesis may increase at the expense of granulopoiesis.

EFFECT OF TOXIC AGENTS ON GRANULOPOIESIS

Figure 3 schematically portrays the essential features regulating the rate of granulocyte production. An analogous reasoning process can be used in dissecting the effect of a toxic agent on granulopoiesis, as has been done with erythropoiesis. Earlier it was mentioned that measurement of granulocyte life-span was impractical in man and animals. Logic tells us that a diminution in concentration of granulocytes in blood is due to either a greater rate of loss from the blood or a reduced input into the blood. In the preantibiotic days, during the course of severe lobar pneumonia the demand for granulocytes on occasion exceeded the ability of the bone marrow to produce enough cells. After the initial granulocytosis, the counts in the blood would fall, immature cells appear, and perusal of the bone marrow would show a marked depletion of mature and proliferating granulocyte precursors. The bone marrow has a large but limited capacity for production of granulocytes, but can be overwhelmed.

Occasionally a drug like phenylbutazone (Butazolidin) will block the transit of cells from the myelocyte to the maturation and storage compartment. The peripheral blood granulocyte count drops to near zero levels. Examination of the bone marrow shows almost complete depletion of metamyelocytes, band and segmented neutrophils. Withdrawal of the drug is almost always followed by repletion of the maturation and storage pool and reappearance of granulocytes in the blood.

Ionizing radiation in sufficient whole body doses to mammals results in a kill of the PSC proportionate to the dose of radiation and a similar kill of the early progenitors (CFU-C) of granulocytes. The identifiable granulocytic precursors are relatively radioresistant and continue to proliferate and mature, thus diminishing in number followed by a peripheral granulopenia.

If a toxic agent represses the genes for production of CSF, lactoferrin, labile granulocytic inhibitor, one would anticipate alterations in the rate of production of granulocytes proportionate to the change in the molecular regulators. Whether this in fact occurs has not been conclusively demonstrated.

LEUKEMOGENESIS BY TOXIC AGENTS

It has long been believed without proof that the target cell for leukemogenesis is the PSC. Fialkow and associates (32) clearly demonstrated, using glucose-6-phosphate dehydrogenase (G6PD) as a marker, that several human hematologic diseases are clonal and arise at the PSC level. Because the G6PD locus is on the X chromosome and only one of the two X's is active in each female somatic cell, women who are heterozygous for the usual B-G6PD gene (Gd^B) and a variant such as Gd^A have two cell populations; in one population Gd^B is active and B-type enzyme is made and in the other, Gd^A is active and A-type G6PD is synthesized. The two enzymes can be distinguished electrophoretically. A tumor with a unicellular origin begins either in a Gd^B cell or in a Gd^A cell. All the neoplastic cells have A or B enzymes, and normal tissues have A and B enzymes. Chronic granulocytic leukemia (CGL) is a monoclonal disease at diagnosis. Many cells may have been initially altered ("preleukemic"), but a single clone evolves into CGL. Single enzymes have been found in platelets, monocytes, eosinophils, and B lymphocytes of several patients with CGL. This, coupled with the presence of the Ph chromosome in granulocytic, erythrocytic, and megakaryocytic cells, proves this disease to have originated from an aberration of a PSC but not necessarily one with self-renewal capacity. Similar studies have shown that *polycythemia vera*, essential thrombocythemia, and agnogenic myeloid metaplasia also arise from a multipotential stem cell.

Acute myeloblastic leukemia (AML) is clearly a clonal disease (of 9 patients studied 4 had B-G6PD and 5 had A-G6PD). In 6 patients with AML that have been studied, double-enzyme phenotypes were found in red cells and in red cell precursors grown *in vitro*, whereas the blast cells, diagnostic of AML, showed a single G6PD. Other studies have shown that AML invokes cells with multipotent differentiative expression, and in others it invokes progenitors with differentiation limited to the granulocytic pathway. The patients in whom multipotent differentiation was found were elderly, whereas those with restrictive differentiation were young. Thus, with human disease, the target cell may be the PSC, an early granulocytic, or lymphocytic (B or T) progenitor.

Leukemia and other malignant diseases have one characteristic in common—non-steady-state growth. Most of the time there is exponential growth in which the growth rate exceeds the death rate. As discussed earlier, some leukemias have clearly originated in a pluripotent cell since either a common cytogenetic abnormality or isoenzyme is found in all hemopoietic cell lines. This does prove that the cell of origin was pluripotent, leaving open the question of whether it was also a high-capacity self-renewing stem cell. Other leukemias, as discussed earlier, arise from cells with limited differentiative ability. Thus it would appear that activation of the "oncogene" for leukemogenesis may take place at different levels in the continuum from the high-capacity self-renewing stem cell through all of the proliferating stages described earlier. On the basis of current knowledge and concepts in experimental leukemogenesis, one can make a plausible argument for assaying the whole continuum of cells from the high-capacity self-renewing stem cell through the pluripotent, tripotent, bipotent, and monopotent progenitors.

In toxicological studies on leukemogenesis in mice, one might profitably avail oneself of a cross between mice that possess different phosphoglycerate kinases (PGK-1). The C3H has PGK-1A and the CBA/Ca has PGK-1B (11). A cross between the C3H and CBA/Ca carries the A and B alleles on the X chromosome. The alleles differ in electrophoretic mobility. The CBA/Ca mouse develops a high incidence of acute myeloblastic leukemia after whole body irradiation as does the C3H mouse. It is likely that the cross will also have a low spontaneous incidence of induced leukemia. If this be the case in the female cross, one could profitably explore the effect of diverse leukemogenic agents and determine if the leukemias in the mouse are monoclonal and identify the target cell(s).

The effects of toxic agents on all tissues and functions are of great importance. Of considerable concern to the public is induction of leukemia. In evaluating whether an agent has a leukemogenic effect, one must select mouse strains with care. For example, if one is interested in the possibility that an agent will activate a leukemogenic virus, the C57Bl/6J male mouse may be the best test animal. It is known to harbor a retrovirus that will produce thymic lymphomata after irradiation of the mouse. In addition, the lifetime spontaneous incidence of thymoma is very low. Furthermore, it has been shown that exposure to benzene 300 ppm, 6 hours per day, 5 days per week for 16 weeks will significantly increase the incidence of thymic lymphomata (22).

If one wishes to test for the potential to produce AML, a suitable mouse strain is the CBA/CaJ male mouse, which has a very low spontaneous incidence of AML but when exposed to 200 to 300 R radiation develops 20% to 30% AML during a lifetime.

The criteria of importance in selecting an inbred mouse for leukemogenesis are:

1. A low spontaneous lifetime incidence—preferably less than 1% of the type of leukemia in which one is interested.

2. Low incidence of other neoplastic disease to minimize competing causes of death and/or morbidity.

3. A known responsiveness to at least one leukemogenic insult.

REFERENCES

1. Ashby, M. (1919): Determination of length of life of transfused blood corpuscles in man. *J. Exp. Med.*, 29:267.
2. Axelrad, A., Croizat, H., Eskinazi, D., Stewart, S., Vaithilingham, D., and vander Gaag, H. (1983): Genetic regulation of DNA synthesis in early erythrocytic progenitors. In: *Hemopoietic*

Stem Cells, edited by S-A. Killmann, E. P. Cronkite, and C. N. Muller-Berat, pp. 238–263, Munksgaard, Copenhagen.

3. Axelrad, A. A., McLeod, D. L., Shreeve, M. M., and Heath, D. S. (1973): Properties of cells that produce erythrocytic colonies *in vitro*. In: *Proceedings of the Second International Workshop on Hemopoiesis in Culture*, edited by W. A. Robinson, pp. 226–237, Airlie House, VA. [DHEW Pub. No. (NIH) 74–205, 1973].

4. Bagby, G. C., Rigas, V. D., Vandenbark, R. M., and Garewall, A. A. (1981): Interaction of lactoferrin, monocytes and T-lymphocyte subsets in the regulation of steady-state granulopoiesis *in vitro*. *J. Clin. Invest.*, 68:56.

5. Bagby, G. C., Jr., and Bennett, R. M. (1982): Feedback regulation of granulopoiesis: Polymerization of lactoferrin abrogates its ability to inhibit CSA production. *Blood*, 60:108–112.

6. Bagby, G. C., Jr., McCall, E., Bergstrom, K. A., and Burger, D. (1983): A monokine regulates colony-stimulating activity production by vascular endothelial cells. *Blood*, 62:663–668.

7. Becker, A. J., McCulloch, E. A., and Till, J. E. (1963): Cytological demonstration of the clonal nature of spleen colonies derived from transplanted mouse marrow cells. *Nature*, 197:452–454.

8. Bleiberg, I., Liron, M., and Feldman, M. (1965): Reversion by erythropoietin of the suppression of erythroid clones caused by transfusion-induced polycythemia. *Transplantation*, 3:706–710.

9. Botnick, L. E., Hannon, E. C., Obbagy, J., and Hellman, S. (1982): Concise report: The variation of hematopoietic stem cell self-renewal capacity as a function of age: Further evidence for heterogenicity of the stem cell compartment. *Blood*, 60:268–271.

10. Bradley, T. R., and Metcalf, D. (1966): The growth of mouse bone marrow cells *in vitro*. *Aust. J. Exp. Biol. Med. Sci.*, 44:287.

11. Brecher, G., Ansell, J. D., Micklem, H. S., Tijio, J.-H., and Cronkite, E. P. (1982): Special proliferative sites are not needed for seeding and proliferation of transfused bone marrow cells in normal syngeneic mice. *Proc. Natl. Acad. Sci. USA*, 79:5085–5087.

12. Broxmeyer, H. E. (1978): Inhibition *in vivo* of mouse granulopoiesis by cell-free activity derived from human polymorphonuclear neutrophils. *Blood*, 51:889–901.

13. Broxmeyer, H. E. (1979): Lactoferrin acts on Ia-like antigen-positive subpopulations of human monocytes to inhibit production of colony stimulatory activity *in vitro*. *J. Clin. Invest.*, 64:1717–1720.

14. Broxmeyer, H. E. (1982): Concise report: Acidic isoferritins and E-type prostaglandins in sources of colony stimulating factors mask detection of cycling granulocyte-macrophage progenitor cells. *Blood*, 60:1042–1045.

15. Broxmeyer, H. E., Bognacki, J., Ralph, P., Dorner, M. H., Lu, L., and Castro-Malaspina, H. (1982): Monocyte-macrophage-derived acidic isoferritins: Normal feedback regulators of granulocyte-macrophage progenitor cells *in vitro*. *Blood*, 60:595–607.

16. Broxmeyer, H. E., DeSousa, M., Smithyman, A., Ralph, P., Hamilton, J., Kurland, J. I., and Bognacki, J. (1980): Specificity and modulation of the action of lactoferrin, a negative feedback regulator of myelopoiesis. *Blood*, 55:324–333.

17. Broxmeyer, H. E., Smithyman, A., Eger, R. R., Meyers, P. A., and DeSousa, M. (1978): Identification of lactoferrin as the granulocyte-derived inhibitor of colony-stimulating activity production. *J. Exp. Med.*, 148:1052–1067.

18. Burlington, H., Cronkite, E. P., Heldman, B., Pappas, N., and Shadduck, R. K. (1983): Tumor-induced granulopoiesis unrelated to colony-stimulating factor. *Blood*, 62:693–696.

19. Cartwright, G. E., Athens, J. W., and Wintrobe, M. M. (1964): The kinetics of granulopoiesis in normal man. *Blood*, 24:780–803.

20. Chertkov, J. L., and Drize, N. J. (1984): Cells forming spleen colonies at 7 or 11 days after injection have different proliferation rates. *Cell Tissue Kinet.*, 17:247–252.

21. Cronkite, E. P., Bond, V. P., Fliedner, T. M., and Killmann, S.-A. (1960): The use of tritiated thymidine in the study of haemopoietic cell proliferation. In: *Ciba Foundation Symposium on Haemopoiesis*, edited by G. E. W. Wolstenholme and M. O'Connor, Churchill, Ltd., London.

22. Cronkite, E. P., Bullis, J. E., Inoue, T., and Drew, R. T. (1984): Benzene inhalation produces leukemia in mice. *Toxicol. Appl. Pharmacol.*, 75: (in press).

23. Cronkite, E. P., Burlington, H., Chanana, A. D., Joel, D. D., Reincke, U., and Stevens, J. (1977): Concepts and observations on the regulation of granulopoiesis. In: *Experimental Hematology Today*, edited by S. J. Baum and G. D. Ledney, pp. 41–48, Springer-Verlag, New York.

24. Cronkite, E. P., Harigaya, K., Garnett, H., Miller, M. E., Honikel, L., and Shadduck, R. K. (1982): Production of colony-stimulating factor by murine bone marrow cell line derived from

the Dexter adherent layer and other properties of this cell line. In: *Experimental Hematology Today 1982*, edited by S. J. Baum, G. D. Ledney, and S. Thierfelder, pp. 11–18, Karger, Basel.

25. Cronkite, E. P., Miller, M. E., Garnett, H., and Harigaya, K. (1983): Regulation of hemopoiesis: Inhibitors and stimulators produced by a murine bone stromal cell line (H-1). In: *Haemopoietic Stem Cells, Alfred Benzon Symposium 18*, edited by Sv.-Aa. Killmann, E. P. Cronkite, and C. N. Muller-Berat, pp. 266–284, Munksgaard, Copenhagen.

26. Cronkite, E. P., and Vincent, P. C. (1969): Granulocytopoiesis. *Ser. Haemat. II*, 3–45.

27. Dancey, J. T., Deubelbeiss, K. A., Harker, L. A., and Finch, C. A. (1976): Neutrophil kinetics in man. *J. Clin. Invest.*, 58:705–715.

28. Deubelbeiss, K. A., Dancey, J. T., Harker, L. A., and Finch, C. A. (1975): Neutrophil kinetics in the dog. *J. Clin. Invest.*, 55:833–839.

29. Dresch, C., Najean, Y., and Bauchet, J. (1975): Kinetic studies of ^{51}Cr and ^{32}P-DFP labeling of granulocytes. *Br. J. Haemat.*, 29:67–78.

30. Fauser, A. A., and Messner, H. A. (1979): Concise report: Proliferative state of human pluripotent hemopoietic progenitors (CFU-GEMM) in normal individuals and under regenerative conditions after bone marrow transplantation. *Blood*, 54:1197–1200.

31. Fauser, A. A., Messner, H. A., Lusis, A. J., and Golde, D. W. (1981): Stimulatory activity for human pluripotent hemopoietic progenitors produced by a human T-lymphocyte cell line. *Stem Cells*, 1:73–80.

32. Fialkow, P. J. (1983): Hierarchical hematologic stem cell relationships studied with glucose-6-phosphate dehydrogenase enzymes. In: *Hematopoietic Stem Cells*, edited by S.-A. Killmann, E. P. Cronkite, and C. N. Muller-Berat, pp. 174–186, Munksgaard, Copenhagen.

33. Fliedner, T. M., Cronkite, E. P., Killmann, S.-A., and Bond, V. P. (1964): Granulocytopoiesis II. Emergence and pattern of labeling of neutrophilic granulocytes in human beings. *Blood*, 24:683–700.

34. Fliedner, T. M., Cronkite, E. P., and Robertson, J. S. (1964): Granulocytopoiesis I. Senescence and random loss of neutrophilic granulocytes in human beings. *Blood*, 24:402–414.

35. Garnett, H. M., Cronkite, E. P., and Harigaya, K. (1982): Regulation of the colony-stimulating activity produced by a murine marrow-derived cell line (H-1). *Proc. Natl. Acad. Sci. USA*, 79:1545–1548.

36. Garnett, H. M., Harigaya, K., and Cronkite, E. P. (1982): Characterization of a murine cell-line derived from cultured bone marrow stromal cells. *Stem Cells*, 2:11–23.

37. Garnett, H. M., Harigaya, K., and Cronkite, E. P. (1984): Influence of a fibroblastoid cell line derived from murine bone marrow (H-1 cells) on stem cell proliferation. *Proc. Soc. Exp. Biol. Med.*, 175:70–73.

38. Gordon, A. S., Neri, R. O., Siegel, C. D., Dornfest, B. S., Hangler, E. S., OcBue, J., and Eisler, M. (1960): Evidence for a circulating leukocytosis-inducing factor (LIF). *Acta Haematol. (Basel)*, 23:323–341.

39. Gray, S. J., and Sterling, K. (1950): Tagging of red cells and plasma proteins with radioactive chromium. *J. Clin. Invest.*, 29:1604–1613.

40. Gregory, C. J., and Henkelman, R. M. (1977): Relationship between early progenitor cells determined by correlation analysis in spleen colonies. In: *Experimental Hematology Today*, edited by S. J. Baum, and G. D. Ledney, pp. 93–110, Springer-Verlag, New York.

41. Hagan, M. P., and MacVittie, T. J. (1981): CFUs kinetics observed *in vivo* by bromodeoxyuridine and near-UV light treatment. *Exp. Hematol.*, 9:123–128.

42. Hara. H. (1980): Kinetics of pluripotent hemopoietic precursors *in vitro* after erythropoietic stimulation or suppression. *Exp. Hematol.*, 8:345–350.

43. Hara, H., and Ogawa, M. (1977): Erythropoietic precursors in mice under erythropoietic stimulation and suppression. *Exp. Hematol.*, 5:141–148.

44. Harigaya, K., Cronkite, E. P., Miller, M. E., and Shadduck, R. K. (1981): Murine bone marrow cell line producing colony-stimulating factor. *Proc. Natl. Acad. Sci. USA*, 78:6963–6966.

45. Harris, R. A., Hogarth, P. M., Wadeson, L. J., Collins, P., McKenzie, I. F. C., and Penington, D. G. (1984): An antigenic difference between cells forming early and late haematopoietic spleen colonies (CFU-S). *Nature*, 307:638–641.

46. Hellman, S., Botnick, L. E., Hannon, E. C., and Vigneulle, R. M. (1978): Proliferative capacity of murine hematopoietic stem cells. *Proc. Natl. Acad. Sci. USA*, 75:490–494.

47. Hesketh, P. J., Sullivan, R., Valeri, C. R., and McCarroll, L. A. (1984): The production of

granulocyte-monocyte colony-stimulating activity by isolated human T lymphocyte subpopulations. *Blood*, 63:1141–1146.

48. Hodgson, G. S., and Bradley, T. R. (1979): Properties of haematopoietic stem cells surviving 5-fluorouracil treatment: evidence for a pre-CFU-S-cell? *Nature*, 281:381–382.
49. Inoue, T., Bullis, J. E., Cronkite, E. P., and Hubner, G. E. (1983): Relationship between number of spleen colonies and ^{125}IdUrd incorporation into spleen and femur. *Proc. Natl. Acad. Sci. USA*, 80:435–438.
50. Inoue, T., and Cronkite, E. P. (1983): The influence of *in vivo* incubation of aged murine spleen colony-forming units on their proliferative capacity. *Mech. Ageing Dev.*, 23:177–190.
51. Jamuar, M. P., and Cronkite, E. P. (1980): The fate of blood granulocytes. *Exp. Hematol.*, 8:884–894.
52. Kohsaki, M., Noguchi, K., Araki, K., Horikoshi, A., Sloman, J. C., Miyake, T., and Murphy, M. J., Jr. (1983): *In vivo* stimulation of murine granulopoiesis by human urinary extract from patients with aplastic anemia. *Proc. Natl. Acad. Sci. USA*. 80:3802–3806.
53. Kurland, J. I., Broxmeyer, H., Pelus, L. M., Bockman, R. S., and Moore, M. A. S. (1978): Role for monocyte-macrophage-derived colony-stimulating factor and prostaglandin E in the positive and negative feedback control of myeloid stem cell proliferation. *Blood*, 52:388–407.
54. Lanotte, M., Metcalf, D., and Dexter, T. M. (1982): Production of monocyte/macrophage colony-stimulating factor by preadipocyte cell lines derived from murine marrow stroma. *J. Cell. Physiol.*, 112:123–127.
55. Lee, E. W., Kocsis, J. J., and Snyder, R. (1981): The use of ferrokinetics in the study of experimental anemia. *Environ. Health Perspect.*, 39:29–37.
56. Liron, M., and Feldman, M. (1965): The specific suppression of the differentiation of erythroid clones in polycythemic animals. *Transplantation*, 3:509–516.
57. Magli, M. C., Iscove, N. N., and Odartchenko, N. (1982): Transient nature of early haematopoietic spleen colonies. *Nature*, 295:527–529.
58. Maloney, M., and Patt, H. M. (1968): Granulocyte transit from bone marrow to blood. *Blood*, 31:195–201.
59. Maloney, M. A., Weber, C. L., and Patt, H. M. (1963): Myelocyte and metamyelocyte transition in the bone marrow of the dog. *Nature*, 197:150–152.
60. Messner, H. A., Fauser, A. A., Lepine, J., and Martin, M. (1980): Properties of human pluripotent hemopoietic progenitors. *Blood Cells*, 6:595–607.
61. Messner, H. A., Izaguirre, C. A., and Jamal, N. (1981): Identification of T-lymphocytes in human mixed hemopoietic colonies. *Blood*, 58:402–405.
62. Metcalf, D., and Burgess, A. W. (1982): Analysis of progenitor commitment to granulocyte or macrophage production. *J. Cell. Physiol.*, 111:275–283.
63. Miller, M. E., Garcia, J. F., Shiue, G. G., Okula, R. M., and Clemons, G. K. (1983): Humoral regulation of erythropoiesis. In: *Haemopoietic Stem Cells, Alfred Benzon Symposium 18*, edited by Sv.-Aa. Killmann, E. P. Cronkite, and C. N. Muller-Berat, pp. 218–288, Munksgaard, Copenhagen.
64. Monette, F. C., and DeMellow, J. B. (1979): The relationship between stem cell seeding efficiency and position in cell cycle. *Cell Tissue Kinet.*, 12:161–175.
65. Nakahata, T., Gross, A. J., and Ogawa, M. (1982): A stochastic model of self-renewal and commitment to differentiation of the primitive hemopoietic stem cells in culture. *J. Cell. Physiol.*, 113:455–458.
66. Patt, H. M., and Maloney, M. (1964): A model of granulocyte kinetics. *Ann. NY Acad. Sci.*, 113:515–522.
67. Patt, H. M., Maloney, M. A., and Lamela, R. A. (1980): Hematopoietic stem cell proliferative behavior as revealed by bromodeoxyuridine labeling. *Exp. Hematol.*, 8:1075–1079.
68. Pelus, L. M., Broxmeyer, H. E., Kurland, J. I., and Moore, M. A. S. (1979): Regulation of macrophage and granulocyte proliferation. *J. Exp. Med.*, 150:277–292.
69. Pennathur-Das, R., Alpen, E., Vichinsky, E., and Lubin, B. (1984): Evidence for a heterogeneous response to erythropoietin in the CFU-E pool of human bone marrow. *Exp. Hematol.*, 12:31–37.
70. Pluznik, D. H., and Sach, L. (1965): The cloning of normal mast cells in tissue culture. *J. Cell. Comp. Physiol.*, 66:319.
71. Preisler, H. D., and Henderson, E. S. (1971): Effect of suppression of erythropoiesis on hematopoietic stem cells in the mouse. *J. Cell. Physiol.*, 79:103–110.

72. Quesenberry, P. J., and Gimbrone, M. A. (1980): Vascular endothelium as a regulator of granu-lopoiesis: Production of CSA by cultured human endothelial cells. *Blood*, 56:1060–1067.
73. Reincke, U., Brookoff, D., Burlington, H., and Cronkite, E. P. (1979): Forced differentiation of CFU-S by iron-55 erythrocytocide. *Blood Cells*, 5:351–376.
74. Reincke, U., Cronkite, E. P., and Hinkelmann, K. (1976): Volumes and cellularity in populations of hematopoietic clones. *Nouv. Rev. Fr. Hematol.*, 16:255–272.
75. Resegotti, L. (1957): Life cycle of granulocytes and lymphocytes determined by making use of ^{59}Fe-labeled hemin as a tracer. *Acta Physiol. Scand.*, 41:325–339.
76. Rosendaal, M., Hodgson, G. S., and Bradley, T. R. (1976): Haemopoietic stem cells are organised for use on the basis of their generation-age. *Nature*, 264:68–69.
77. Salner, A. L., Obbagy, J. E., and Hellman, S. (1982): Differing stem cell self-renewal of lectin-separated murine bone marrow fractions. *J. Natl. Cancer Inst.*, 68:639–641.
78. Schofield, R., and Lajtha, L. G. (1969): Graft size considerations in the kinetics of spleen colony development. *Cell Tissue Kinet.*, 2:147–155.
79. Shemin, D., and Rittenberg, D. (1946): Life span of human red blood cell. *J. Biol. Chem.*, 166:627.
80. Siminovitch, L., McCulloch, E. A., and Till, J. E. (1963): The distribution of colony-forming cells among spleen colonies. *J. Cell Comp. Physiol.*, 62:327–336.
81. Stanley, E. R., Hanson, G., Woodcock, J., and Metcalf, D. (1975): Colony stimulating factor and the regulation of granulopoiesis and macrophage production. *Fed. Proc.*, 34:2272–2278.
82. Stephenson, J. R., Axelrad, A. A., McCloud, D. C., and Shreeve, M. M. (1971): Induction of colonies of hemoglobin synthesizing cells by erythropoietin *in vitro*. *Proc. Natl. Acad. Sci. USA*, 68:1542–1546.
83. Stryckmans, P., Cronkite, E. P., Fache, J., Fliedner, T. M., and Ramos, J. (1966): Deoxyribonu-cleic acid synthesis time of erythropoietic cells in human beings. *Nature (Lond.)*, 211:717–720.
84. Till, J. E., and McCulloch, E. A. (1961): A direct measurement of the radiation sensitivity of normal mouse bone marrow cells. *Radiat. Res.*, 14:213–222.
85. Till, J. E., McCulloch, E. A., and Siminovitch, L. (1964): A stochastic model of stem cell proliferation, based on the growth of spleen colony-forming cells. *Proc. Natl. Acad. Sci. USA*, 51:29–36.
86. Vogel, H., Niewisch, H., and Matiolo, G. (1968): The self-renewal probability of hemopoietic stem cells. *J. Cell. Physiol.*, 72:221–228.

Toxicology of the Blood and Bone Marrow,
edited by Richard D. Irons. Raven Press,
New York © 1985.

Chemical Toxicity of the Erythrocyte

Ernest Beutler

*Scripps Clinic and Research Foundation, Department of Basic and Clinical Research,
Division of Hematology/Oncology, La Jolla, California 92037*

Each day the bone marrow produces more than 10^{11} blood cells. Circulating in the bloodstream, these cells live for an average of approximately 120 days and then are removed from the bloodstream by the reticuloendothelial system. The red cell possesses effective mechanisms for cell repair when it is damaged in the circulation, although it does not contain a nucleus and is therefore unable to synthesize new proteins. But defenses against some insults appear to be insufficient to permit the cell to continue to circulate. It is sometimes removed long before it has lived out its expected life of 120 days, or even undergoes lysis in the bloodstream.

Although the mechanisms of normal red cell senescence have been studied extensively for several decades, we do not yet understand why the cell is removed after circulating for 120 days. Often the mechanism by which toxins shorten the red cell life-span is also not well understood. Among the explanations that have been proposed, and those that are most likely to be correct, are (a) loss in deformability of the cell brought about either by changes in the membrane, such as the cross-linking of membrane proteins, or by changes in internal viscosity resulting from water loss and (b) the attachment of immunoglobulins to the red cell membrane, leading to phagocytosis of erythrocytes. The effect of toxins on red cell life-span may be exerted by simulating the aging of red cells, making a young erythrocyte appear old to the cells that remove it from the circulation.

RED CELL DESTRUCTION BY ANTIBODIES

The attachment of antibodies to a red cell may abruptly terminate its life. Three different mechanisms may lead to red cell destruction. The IgM antibodies fix complement on the erythrocyte surface, and even a relatively small amount of antibody will lead to its lysis by complement. Agglutination of erythrocytes into large masses may also occur, particularly with IgM antibodies, resulting in the sequestration of red cells in capillaries through which they can no longer pass. Perhaps most important is the effect both of complement components and of the Fc receptor of immunoglobulin molecules clustered on the surface of the cell on phagocytes. Erythrocytes that have been sensitized in this way do not easily pass the macrophages that guard the sinusoids of spleen, liver, and bone marrow.

Phagocytes are activated by the C3b fragment of complement and by aggregated Fc receptors and will engulf red cells.

Usually when antibodies are involved in the destruction of red blood cells their appearance is not related to the administration of drugs. For example, when a patient is transfused with red cells having antigens on their surface that are foreign to the recipient, antibody-mediated red cell destruction may occur. Hemolysis may also be the result of the elaboration of "forbidden" antibodies by a patient against his own red cells either because of the development of a benign autoimmune disorder, or because of the development of a malignant clone of cells, as in chronic lymphocytic leukemia or one of the lymphomas.

Occasionally, however, the administration of drugs plays an essential role in the development of antibody-mediated hemolytic anemia. Three mechanisms of drug-mediated hemolysis have been delineated. The first of these to have been described is that caused by the antimonial stibophen (32). The mechanism that results in red cell injury has been designated the "immune complex mechanism" or the "innocent bystander phenomenon." The IgM antibodies directed against the drug or perhaps drug-protein complexes form immune complexes in the plasma. These complexes bind reversibly to red cells and may induce activation and binding of complement components to the red cell membrane. It is characteristic of this mechanism that the antibodies have no affinity for the red cell itself, and the drug is not bound to the membrane. Drugs that have caused hemolytic anemia through this mechanism are listed in Table 1.

A second mechanism through which drugs induce immune-mediated hemolytic anemia involves the firm binding of the drug to the red cell surface. Penicillin-induced hemolysis is a prototype of this kind of reaction. The IgM antibodies that are commonly directed against penicillin do not play a role in this type of reaction. Rather, it is the less common IgG antibodies directed against the benzylpenicilloyl determinant of penicillin that are usually responsible for hemolysis. Occasionally, drugs other than penicillin may be involved in this type of reaction. Such drugs are listed in Table 2.

One of the most interesting drug-related types of hemolytic anemia is caused by methyldopa, L-DOPA, and mefenamic acid. Here antibodies are not formed against the drug at all. Rather, they are formed against common red cell antigens, usually determinants of the Rh complex. The antibodies are ordinarily of the IgG variety. Interestingly, a high proportion of patients taking methyldopa develop a positive direct antiglobulin test, with an estimated frequency varying from 8% to 36%.

TABLE 1. *Drugs that have caused hemolytic anemia by means of the immune complex mechanism*

Quinine (55)	Rifampicin (44)
Quinidine (17,24)	Antazoline (6)
Stibophen (32)	Methotrexate (80)
Chlorpropamide (48)	

TABLE 2. *Drugs that have caused hemolytic anemia by means of firm binding of drug to red cell membrane*

Penicillin (46,62,70,75,79)	Tetracycline (77)
Cephalosporins (29)	Carbromal (68)

However, only a small percentage of the patients who develop detectable immunoglobulin on their red cells actually develop hemolytic anemia. The mechanism of this type of hemolytic reaction is not understood. It appears that in some way these drugs interfere with normal immune recognition. It has been proposed that the drug may interact with human T lymphocytes, resulting in a loss of suppressor function (42).

OXIDATIVE DAMAGE TO RED CELLS

One of the principal functions of red cells is the delivery of oxygen from the lungs to the tissues. When firmly bound to heme in a hydrophobic crevice in the hemoglobin molecule, the oxygen is harmless enough, but a relatively high concentration of free molecular oxygen is dissolved in the red cell water. Moreover, as the oxygen molecule is extracted from hemoglobin, highly reactive oxygen species such as the superoxide anion may arise (12). The presence of such reactive species has the capacity to initiate lipid peroxidation in the red cell membrane, to inactivate vital red cell enzymes, and to denature the hemoglobin molecule itself.

Red cells have a number of defense mechanisms against activated oxygen attack. Catalase decomposes hydrogen peroxide to water. Reduced glutathione also protects against oxidative attack. Through the enzyme glutathione peroxidase, glutathione reduces even very low levels of hydrogen peroxide. In addition, an enzyme yet to be characterized utilizes glutathione to protect membrane lipids against peroxidation (26). The most clinically important enzyme in the defense of red cells against oxidative attack is glucose-6-phosphate dehydrogenase (G6PD) (7).

The administration of certain drugs, commonly designated as "oxidant" compounds, increases the generation of activated oxygen species and may overwhelm the defense mechanisms of the cell. This is particularly likely to occur when the defenses of the erythrocyte are already defective owing to a hereditary enzyme deficiency. Although it is likely that most of the drugs known to produce hemolytic anemia in susceptible individuals can damage and destroy normal erythrocytes, hemolytic anemia due to most of these compounds is oberved only in persons with hereditary enzyme deficiencies. But this is not universally true. Apparently, the defense mechanisms vary considerably in their efficiency in dealing with the effects of drugs. Thus, in the case of some drugs, such as primaquine, the dose required to produce hemolysis of normal red cells is vastly larger than that required to produce hemolysis in enzyme-deficient cells. In the case of other drugs, such as phenylhydrazine, the dose required to destroy normal red cells is only slightly higher than that required for susceptible cells (20).

Extensive lists of drugs and other chemical compounds that have a putative
hemolytic effect when they challenge G6PD-deficient red cells have been published.
A critical analysis of the evidence linking the administration of these compounds
to hemolysis has shown that in many instances the hemolysis even of enzyme-
deficient cells is so mild as to make it quite safe to administer the drug to an
enzyme-deficient individual. Such drugs are listed in Table 3. On the other hand,
there is another group of drugs, well-tolerated by normal subjects, that may produce
severe hemolysis in enzyme-deficient patients. Such drugs are listed in Table 4.

Since the detoxification of active oxygen species seems to require the intervention
of reduced glutathione, enzymatic lesions that impair the reduction of this sulfhydryl

TABLE 3. *Drugs that can probably be given safely in normal
therapeutic doses to G6PD-deficient subjects (without
nonspherocytic hemolytic anemia) [references in (7)]*

Acetaminophen (paracetamol, Tylenol, Tralgon, p-hydroxyacetanilide)	Menapthone
	p-Aminobenzoic acid
	Phenylbutazone
Acetophenetidin (phenacetin)	Phenytoin
Acetylsalicylic acid (aspirin)	Probenecid (Benemid)
Aminopyrine (Pyramidon, amidopyrine)	Procaine amide hydrochloride (Pronestyl)
Antazoline (Antistine)	Pyrimethamine (Daraprim)
Antipyrine	Quinidine
Ascorbic acid (vitamin C)	Quinine
Benzhexol (Artane)	Streptomycin
Chloramphenicol	Sulfacytine
Chlorguanide (Proguanil, Paludrine)	Sulfadiazine
	Sulfaquanidine
Chloroquine	Sulfamerazine
Colchicine	Sulfamethoxypyriazine (Kynex)
Diphenylhydramine (Benedryl)	Sulfisoxazole (Gantrisin)
Isoniazide	Trimethoprim
L-DOPA	Tripelennamine (Pyribenzamine)
Menadione sodium bisulfite (Hykinone)	Vitamin K

TABLE 4. *Drugs and chemicals that have clearly been
shown to cause clinically significant hemolytic anemia in
G6PD deficiency[a]*

Acetanilid	Phenylazodiaminopyridine (pyridium) (73)
Methylene blue	Sulfanilamide
Nalidixic acid (Negram)	Sulfacetamide
Naphthalene	Sulfapyridine
Niridazole (Ambilhar)	Sulfamethoxazole (Gantanol)
Nitrofurantoin (Furadantin)	Thiazolesulfone
Phenylhydrazine	Toluidine blue
Primaquine	Trinitrotoluene (TNT)
Pamaquine	
Pentaquine	

[a]Additional references in ref. 7.

compound have often been thought to be implicated in causing sensitivity to drug-induced hemolysis. The most common enzyme deficiency of red cells, that of G6PD, is the prototype of hereditary sensitivity to hemolytic anemia induced by oxidant drugs. The biochemistry and genetics of G6PD deficiency have been extensively documented (7), and there is no doubt that a lack of this enzyme is associated with increased susceptibility to drug-induced hemolysis. On the other hand, the role of other enzyme deficiencies in drug-induced hemolysis is much less clear. Glutathione reductase, 6-phosphogluconate dehydrogenase, glutathione per-oxidase, γ-glutamyl cysteine synthetase, glutathione synthetase, glutathione S-transferase, catalase, and the glutathione-dependent enzyme, which prevents lipid peroxidation that we have recently described (26), could all be considered essential in protection against drug-induced hemolysis. Surprisingly, however, a deficiency of most of these enzymes has not proven to confer sensitivity to drug-induced hemolysis.

Lowered glutathione reductase activity is usually not due to hereditary abnormalities, but rather to decreased riboflavin intake. Thus, it has been possible to manipulate the activity of this enzyme both in man and in animals and thereby to show that even moderately severe deficiencies of the enzyme do not result in hemolytic anemia (9). In one family, essentially total absence of gluthathione reductase has been described (49). Hemolytic anemia subsequent to exposure to fava beans was observed but there was neither chronic hemolytic anemia, nor was there a history of sensitivity to the hemolytic effect of oxidant drugs. Obviously, compensation for a lack of gluthathione reductase is very efficient.

Equally remarkable is the lack of hematologic effect of a severe deficiency of catalase. Absence of this enzyme has been described both in Japanese (71) and in Swiss (1) populations, but no hemolytic anemia has been observed.

Glutathione peroxidase deficiency also appears to be entirely benign. A modest deficiency of this enzyme occurs as a genetic polymorphism in Mediterranean populations. It is not associated with any demonstrated adverse effect (8). Severe selenium deficiency also results in glutathione peroxidase deficiency, since selenium is a part of the active site of this enzyme. Again, no known adverse hematologic effects have been described (40,72). Although clear-cut clinical descriptions are lacking, a single patient with virtually absent 6-phosphogluconate dehydrogenase appeared to be entirely normal (61). Defects in the enzymes of glutathione synthesis, γ-glutamyl cysteine synthetase, and glutathione synthetase are associated with a severe deficiency of red cell glutathione. This is associated with mild chronic hemolytic anemia, susceptibility to drug-induced hemolysis, and, in at least one instance, sensitivity to the hemolytic effect of fava beans (7).

When enzymatic defenses are competent, normal hemoglobin is able to withstand free-radical and peroxide attack without denaturation for the life-span of the red cell. There are, however, abnormalities of the amino acid sequence of the hemoglobin molecule that result in instability, even in the unstressed state. Such mutations usually involve amino acid residues that are in the region of the molecule that binds heme or may be in those areas in which the subunits interact with each other (37). Such "unstable" hemoglobins gradually denature within the erythrocyte during its life-span, forming insoluble precipitates that are often "pitted" from the erythrocyte in the spleen. Thus, even in the absence of oxidative stress a hemolytic anemia is often present. When "oxidative" drugs are given, the rate of hemolysis may accelerate markedly.

Hemolytic anemia occurring as a result of ingestion of the sulfonamides was the presenting symptom of the first patient found to have hemoglobin Zürich (25). Increased susceptibility to drug-induced hemolysis has been observed subsequently in other patients with unstable hemoglobins, but since these abnormal hemoglobins are relatively rare, the spectrum of drugs that produces hemolysis has not yet been clearly defined. It probably resembles very closely the list presented in Table 4.

HEMOLYTIC ANEMIA DUE TO NONOXIDATIVE DRUGS

A considerable number of chemical compounds other than the oxidative drugs listed in Table 4 have also been associated with nonimmunologically mediated hemolytic anemia. A variety of mechanisms are involved. Arsine gas, formed in the course of many industrial processes, is a well-recognized cause of hemolytic anemia (38). Severe anemia, jaundice, and hemoglobinuria may result from exposure to sufficient amounts of the gas. The mechanism has not been elucidated, but the reactions of arsenic compounds with enzyme sulfhydryl groups and with sulfhydryl groups in the membrane presumably are involved.

Lead has many toxic effects. One of the features of chronic lead intoxication is a modest shortening of red cell life-span (76,78). The mechanism of hemolysis induced by lead is not altogether clear. It is of interest, however, that the metal is a potent inhibitor of the enzyme pyrimidine 5′-nucleotidase (74) and that, as in the hereditary form of this enzyme deficiency, the enzyme deficiency produced by lead poisoning is associated with marked basophilic stippling. In addition, lead interferes with the normal production of erythrocytes. It inhibits several of the enzymes of heme sythesis (33,76).

Copper also produces hemolytic anemia. This may occur as a result of suicide attempts and has also been reported in the course of hemodialysis when the hemodialysis fluid is contaminated by copper from pipes (13,22,43). The high copper levels that occur in ceruloplasmin deficiency (Wilson's disease) also cause hemolytic anemia (19,30,53,66). The mechanism of copper-induced hemolytic anemia has not been elucidated entirely, but a number of red cell enzymes are exquisitely sensitive to inhibition by the metal (10). Hemolytic anemia may be caused by water, as in the accidental infusion of large amounts of water into the systemic circulation or in near-drowning (65). Many chemicals have been reported sporadically to have caused hemolytic anemia. A list of such chemicals is given in Table 5.

Certain venoms are also associated with red cell destruction. Bee stings (18) and spider bites (52,56) have all been associated with hemolytic anemia. Although snake venoms often contain an enzyme that converts lecithin to lysolecithin, which is potently hemolytic *in vitro*, snake bites only rarely produce hemolysis.

TABLE 5. *Chemicals that may cause hemolytic anemia by nonoxidative, nonimmune mechanisms*

Arsine (38,47)	Hyperbaric oxygen (54)
Lead (76,78)	Resourcin (27)
Copper (13,22,43)	Apiol (50)
Chlorate (36)	Nitrobenzine (35)
Salicylazosulphapyridine (39)	Zinc ethylene bisdithiocarbonate (63)
Phenazopyridine (2)	Aniline (51)
Formaldehyde (60)	Mephenisin (64)
p-Aminosalicylic acid (11,14)	d-Penicillamine (34)
Cisplatin (28,45)	

DRUG-INDUCED MEGALOBLASTIC ANEMIA

Certain drugs may cause aplastic anemia by destroying bone marrow stem cells. This type of anemia is described by E. P. Cronkite and C. D. Wilson *(this volume)*. In addition, however, drugs that interfere with DNA synthesis may disturb the maturation of erythroid cells in the marrow and produce a megaloblastic anemia (5). Purine analogs such as 6-mercaptopurine, 6-thioguanine, or azathioprine may have such an effect. Drugs that block the synthesis of pyrimidine nucleotides may also produce a megaloblastic anemia. Included are such drugs as 5-fluoro-2'-deoxyuridine and 6-azauridine. Inhibitors of deoxyribonucleotide synthesis such as hydroxyurea also produce megaloblastic changes. Certain drugs such as phenylhydantoin derivatives and birth control drugs produce a megaloblastic anemia that is responsive to treatment with folic acid. It has been suggested (67) that some of these drugs interfere with the absorption of folate polyglutamates by impairing deconjugation and in this way produce folate deficiency. However, the validity of this interpretation has been questioned (4).

TOXIC METHEMOGLOBINEMIA

In the course of oxygen loading and unloading from the red cell, the iron of heme generally remains in the divalent state. Occasionally, however, even under normal circumstances, an additional electron is lost from the heme so that the iron becomes trivalent. The brown pigment formed is designated methemoglobin, a hemoglobin derivative that is unable to bind oxygen and is therefore physiologically useless. The oxidation of one or more of the hemes of hemoglobin affects, moreover, the ability of the other hemes to release oxygen, producing a left shift in the oxygen dissociation curve. The red cell has a mechanism for dealing with this undesirable state of affairs. Reduced nicotinamide adenine dinucleotide (NADH) formed in the oxidation of glyceraldehyde phosphate to 1,3-diphosphoglyceric acid can reduce cytochrome b_5 through the mediation of the enzyme NADH diaphorase. Reduced cytochrome b_5 delivers its electron to the trivalent iron of heme and reduces it to hemoglobin, which can then again function as an iron-carrying compound. Certain drugs have the capacity to greatly increase the rate at which hemoglobin is converted to methemoglobin, and this may overwhelm the capacity of red cells to reduce the methemoglobin to hemoglobin.

TABLE 6. *Amino and nitro compounds producing methemoglobinemia. See (23) for additional references*

Acetanilid	Nitroglycerin
α Naphylamine	Nitrosobenzene
Aminophenol	p-Aminopropiophenone
Ammonium nitrate	Paranitraniline
Amyl nitrite	Paraquat (58)
Aniline	Phenacetin
Anilinoethanol	Phenezopyridine HCl (15,57)
Benzocaine (59)	Phenylenediamine
Bismuth subnitrate	Phenylhydroxylamine
Butyl nitrite (69)	Prilocaine (21)
Cetrimide (3)	Prontosil
Dimethylamine	Sodium and potassium nitrate (31)
Dinitrobenzene	Sodium nitrite
Ethyl nitrite	Sulfanilamide
Hydroxylacetanilide	Sulfapyridine
Hydroxylamine	Sulfathiazole
Lidocaine (59)	Toluenediamine
Methylacetanilide	Tolylhydroxylamine
Nitrobenzene	Trinitrotoluene

Some of the drugs that produce methemoglobinemia are listed in Table 6. Many chemical compounds, particularly aniline derivatives, are well known to produce methemoglobinemia in man and experimental animals and have been reviewed elsewhere (41). Not surprisingly, it has been found that persons with hereditary impairment of methemoglobin reduction develop higher levels of methemoglobinemia when exposed to drugs than do individuals who have a normal complement of methemoglobin-reducing enzyme (16). In actual practice, however, most patients with drug-induced methemoglobinemia are not heterozygous for NADH diaphorase. Infants are more susceptible to methemoglobinemia than are adults. The capacity of red cells of newborns to reduce methemoglobin is less than that of red cells of adults. Recently, methemoglobinemia associated with diarrhea and acidosis has been observed in infants, but the toxic principle that produces methemoglobinemia in this disorder remains unknown (81).

ACKNOWLEDGMENTS

This work was supported in part by the National Institutes of Health, Division of Heart, Lung, and Blood grant HL25552. This is Publication 3310BCR from the Research Institute of Scripps Clinic.

REFERENCES

1. Aebi, H., Bossi, E., Cantz, M., Matsubara, S., and Suter, H. (1968): Acatalas(em)ia in Switzerland. In: *Hereditary Disorders of Erythrocyte Metabolism*, edited by E. Beutler, pp. 41–65. City of Hope Symposium Series, Vol. I, Grune & Stratton, New York.
2. Ahmad, S. (1980): Hemolytic anemia and hepatitis induced by phenazopyridine. *Arch. Intern. Med.*, 140:1398–1399 (Letter).
3. Baraka, A., Yamut, F., and Wakid, N. (1980): Cetrimide-induced methaemoglobinemia after surgical excision of hydatid cyst. *Lancet*, 2:88–89.

4. Baugh, C. M., and Krumdieck, C. L. (1969): Effects of phenytoin on folic-acid conjugases in man. *Lancet*, 2:519–521.
5. Beck, W. S. (1983): The megaloblastic anemias. In: *Hematology*, edited by W. J. Williams, E. Beutler, A. J. Erslev, and M. A. Lichtman, pp. 434–465, 3d ed., McGraw-Hill, New York.
6. Bengtsson, U., Staffan, A., Aurell, M., and Kaijser, B. (1975): Antazoline-induced immune hemolytic anemia, hemoglobinuria and acute renal failure. *Acta Med. Scand.*, 198:223–227.
7. Beutler, E. (1978): *Hemolytic Anemia in Disorders of Red Cell Metabolism*, Plenum Press, New York.
8. Beutler, E., and Matsumoto, F. (1975): Ethnic variation in red cell glutathione peroxidase activity. *Blood*, 46:103–110.
9. Beutler, E., and Srivastava, S. K. (1970): Relationship between gluthathione reductase activity and drug-induced haemolytic anaemia. *Nature*, 226:759–760.
10. Boulard, M., Blume, K., and Beutler, E. (1972): The effect of copper on red cell enzyme activities. *J. Clin. Invest.*, 51:459–461.
11. Bower, G. (1964): Skin rash, hepatitis, and hemolytic anemia caused by para-aminosalicylic acid. *Am. Rev. Respir. Dis.*, 89:440–443.
12. Carrell, R. W., Winterbourn, C. C., and Rachmilewitz, E. A. (1975): Activated oxygen and haemolysis. *Br. J. Haematol.*, 30:259–264.
13. Chuttani, H. K., Gupta, P. S., Gulati, S., and Gupta, D. N. (1965): Acute copper sulfate poisoning. *Am. J. Med.*, 39:849–854.
14. Claps, F. X. (1957): Two cases of methemoglobinemia and acute hemolytic anemia with death following the ingestion of a solution of para-aminosalicylic acid. *Am. Rev. Tb. Pulm. Dis.*, 76:862–866.
15. Cohen, B. L., and Bovasso, G. J., Jr. (1971): Acquired methemoglobinemia and hemolytic anemia following excessive pyridium (phenazopyridine hydrochloride) ingestion. *Clin. Pediatr.*, 10:537–540.
16. Cohen, R. J., Sachs, J. R., Wicker, D. J., and Conrad, M. E. (1968): Methemoglobinemia provoked by malarial chemoprophylaxis in Vietnam. *N. Engl. J. Med.*, 279:1127–1131.
17. Croft Jr., J. D., Swisher, S. N., Gilliland, B. C., Bakemeier, R. F., Leddy, J. P., and Weed, R. I. (1968): Coombs test positivity induced by drugs: Mechanisms of immunologic reactions and red cell destruction. *Ann. Intern. Med.*, 68:176.
18. Dacie, J. V. (1967): *The Haemolytic Anaemias* p. 1091, Grune & Stratton, New York, 2nd ed.
19. Deiss, A., Lee, G. R., and Cartwright, G. E. (1970): Hemolytic anemia in Wilson's disease. *Ann. Intern. Med.*, 73:413–418.
20. Dern, R. J., Beutler, E., and Alving, A. S. (1955): The hemolytic effect of primaquine. V. Primaquine sensitivity as a manifestation of a multiple drug sensitivity. *J. Lab. Clin. Med.*, 45:40–50.
21. Duncan, P. G., and Kobrinsky, N. (1983): Prilocaine-induced methemoglobinemia in a newborn infant. *Anesthesiology*, 59:75–76.
22. Fairbanks, V. F. (1967): Copper sulfate-induced hemolytic anemia. *Arch. Intern. Med.*, 120:428–432.
23. Finch, C. A. (1948): Methemoglobinemia and sulfhemoglobinemia. *N. Engl. J. Med.*, 239:470–478.
24. Freedman, A. L., Barr, P. S., and Brody, E. (1956): Hemolytic anemia due to quinidine: Observations on its mechanism. *Am. J. Med.*, 20:806.
25. Frick, P. G., Hitzig, W. H., and Betke, K. (1962): Hemoglobin Zurich. I. A new hemoglobin anomaly associated with acute hemolytic episodes with inclusion bodies after sulfonamide therapy. *Blood*, 20:261–271.
26. Fujii, S., Dale, G., and Beutler, E. (1984): Glutathione-dependent protection against the oxidative damage of human red cell membrane. *Blood*, 63:1096.
27. Gasser, V. C. (1954): Perakute haemolytische Innenkoerperanamie mit Methaemoglobinamie nach Behandlung eines Saeuglingsekzems mit Resorcin. *Helv. Paediatr. Acta*, 9:285–297.
28. Getaz, E. P., Beckley, S., Fitzpatrick, J., and Dozier, A. (1980): Cisplatin-induced hemolysis. *N. Engl. J. Med.*, 302:334–335.
29. Gralnick, H. R., McGinniss, M., Elton, W., and McCurdy, P. (1971): Hemolytic anemia associated with cephalothin. *JAMA*, 217:1193–1197.
30. Hamlyn, A. N., Gollan, J. L., Douglas, A. P., and Sherlock, S. (1977): Fulminant Wilson's disease

with haemolysis and renal failure: Copper studies and assessment of dialysis regimens. *Br. Med. J.*, 2:660–663.

31. Harris, J. C., Rumack, B. H., Peterson, R. G., and McGuire, B. M. (1979): Methemoglobinemia resulting from absorption of nitrates. *JAMA*, 242:2869–2871.

32. Harris, J. W. (1956): Studies on the mechanism of drug-induced hemolytic anemia. *J. Lab. Clin. Med.*, 47:760–775.

33. Harris J. W., and Kellermeyer, R. W. (1970): Acquired abnormality: Porphyrinuria. In: *The Red Cell*, pp. 35–63. Harvard University Press, Cambridge, Mass.

34. Harrison, E. E., and Hickman, J. W. (1976): D-penicillamine and haemolytic anaemia. *Lancet*, 1:38.

35. Hunter, D. (1943): Industrial toxicology. *Q. J. Med.*, 12:185–258.

36. Jackson, R. C., Elder, W. J., and McDonnell, H. (1961): Sodium-chlorate poisoning complicated by acute renal failure. *Lancet*, 2:1381–1383.

37. Jacob, H. S., Brain, M. C., Dacie, J. V., Carrell, R. W., and Lehmann, H. (1968): Abnormal haem binding and globin SH group blockade in unstable haemoglobins. *Nature*, 218:1214–1217.

38. Jenkins, G. C., Ind, J. E., Kazantzis, G., and Owen, R. (1965): Arsine poisoning: Massive haemolysis with minimal impairment of renal function. *Br. Med. J.*, 2:78–80.

39. Kaplinsky, N., and Frankl, O. (1978): Salicylazosulphapyridine-induced heinz body anemia. *Acta Haematol.*, 59:310–314.

40. Kien, C. L., and Ganther, H. E. (1983): Manifestations of chronic selenium deficiency in a child receiving total parenteral nutrition. *Am. J. Clin. Nutr.*, 37:319–328.

41. Kiese, M. (1966): The biochemical production of ferrihemoglobin-forming derivatives from aromatic amines, and mechanisms of ferrihemoglobin formation. *Pharmacol. Rev.*, 18:1091–1161.

42. Kirtland, H. K. III, Mohler, D. N., and Horowitz, D. (1980): Methyldopa inhibition of suppressor-lymphocyte function. A proposed cause of autoimmune hemolytic anemia. *N. Engl. J. Med.*, 302:825–832.

43. Klein, W. J. Jr., Metz, E. N., and Price, A. R. (1972): Acute copper intoxication. A hazard of hemodialysis. *Arch. Intern. Med.*, 129:578–582.

44. Lakshminarayan, S., Sahn, S. A., and Hudson, L. D. (1973): Massive haemolysis caused by rifampicin. *Br. Med. J.*, 2:282–283.

45. Levi, J. A., Aroney, R. S., and Dalley, D. N. (1981): Haemolytic anaemia after cisplatin treatment. *Br. Med. J.*, 282:2003–2004.

46. Levine, B., and Redmond, A. (1967): Immunochemical mechanisms of penicillin induced Coombs positivity and hemolytic anemia in man. *Int. Arch. Allergy Appl. Immunol.*, 31:594–606.

47. Levinsky, W. J., Smalley, R. V., Hillyer, P. N., and Shindler, R. L. (1970): Arsine hemolysis. *Arch. Environ. Health*, 20:436–439.

48. Logue, G. L., Boyd, A. E., and Rosse, W. F. (1970): Chlorpropamide-induced immune hemolytic anemia. *N. Engl. J. Med.*, 283:900–904.

49. Loos, H., Roos, D., Weening, R., and Houwerzijl, J. (1976): Familial deficiency of glutathione reductase in human blood cells. *Blood*, 48:53–62.

50. Lowenstein, L., and Ballew, D. H. (1958): Fatal acute haemolytic anaemia, thrombocytopenic purpura, nephrosis and hepatitis resulting from ingestion of a compound containing apiol. *Can. Med. Assoc. J.*, 78:195–198.

51. Lubash, G. D., Phillips, R. E., Shields, J. D., and Bonsnes, R. W. (1964): Acute aniline poisoning treated by hemodialysis. *Arch. Intern. Med.*, 114:530–532.

52. Madrigal, G. C., Ercolani, R. L., and Wenzl, J. E. (1972): Toxicity from a bite of the brown spider (loxosceles reclusus) skin necrosis, hemolytic anemia, and hemoglobinuria in a nine-year-old child. *Clin. Pediatr.*, 11:641–644.

53. McIntyre, N., Clink, H. M., Levi, A. J., Cumings, J. N., and Sherlock, S. (1967): Hemolytic anemia in Wilson's disease. *N. Engl. J. Med.*, 276:439–444.

54. Mengel, C. E., Kann, H. E. Jr., Heyman, A., and Metz, E. (1965): Effects of in vivo hyperoxia on erythrocytes. II. Hemolysis in a human after exposure to oxygen under high pressure. *Blood*, 25:822–829.

55. Muirhead, E. E., Halden, E. R., and Granes, M. (1958): Drug dependent Coombs (antiglobulin) test and anemia: Observations on quinine and acetophenetidine (phenacetin). *Arch. Intern. Med.*, 101:87–96.

56. Nance, W. E. (1961): Hemolytic anemia of necrotic arachnidism. *Am. J. Med.*, 31:801–807.

57. Nathan, D. M., Siegel, A. J., and Bunn, H. F. (1977): Acute methemoglobinemia and hemolytic anemia with phenazopyridine. *Arch. Intern. Med.*, 137:1636–1638.
58. Ng, L. L., Naik, R. B., and Polak, A. (1982): Paraquat ingestion with methaemoglobinaemia treated with methylene blue. *Br. Med. J.*, 284:1445–1446.
59. O'Donohue, W. J., Moss, L. M., and Angelillo, V. A. (1980): Acute methemoglobinemia induced by topical Benzocaine and Lidocaine. *Arch. Intern. Med.*, 140:1508–1509.
60. Orringer, E. P., and Mattern, W. D. (1976): Formaldehyde-induced hemolysis during chronic hemodialysis. *N. Engl. J. Med.*, 294:1416–1420.
61. Parr, C. W., and Fitch, L. I. (1967): Inherited quantitative variations of human phosphogluconate dehydrogenase. *Ann. Hum. Genet.*, 30:339–353.
62. Petz, L. D., and Fudenberg, H. H. (1966): Coombs-positive hemolytic anemia caused by penicillin administration. *N. Engl. J. Med.*, 274:171–178.
63. Pinkhas, J., Djaldetti, M., Joshua, H., Resnick, C., and Tschirren, B. (1963): Sulfhemoglobinemia and acute hemolytic anemia with Heinz bodies following contact with a fungicide-zinc ethylene bisidithiocarbamate in subject with glucose-6-phosphate dehydrogenase deficiency and hypocatalasemia. *Blood*, 21:484–494.
64. Pugh, J. I., and Enderby, G. E. H. (1947): Haemoglobinuria after intravenous myanesin. *Lancet*, 2:387–388.
65. Rath, C. E. (1953): Drowning hemoglobinuria. *Blood*, 8:1099–1104.
66. Roche-Sicot, J., and Benhamou, J.-P. (1977): Acute intravascular hemolysis and acute liver failure associated as a first manifestation of Wilson's disease. *Ann. Intern. Med.*, 86:301–303.
67. Rosenberg, I. H., Streiff, R. R., Godwin, H. A., and Castle, W. B. (1968): Impairment of intestinal deconjugation of dietary folate. A possible explanation of megaloblastic anemia associated with phenytoin therapy. *Lancet*, 2:530–532.
68. Stefanini, M., and Johnson, N. L. (1970): Positive antihuman globulin test in patients receiving carbromal. *Am. J. Med. Sci.*, 259:49–55.
69. Steiner, R. W., and Manoguerra, A. S. (1980): Butyl nitrite and methemoglobinemia. *Ann. Intern. Med.*, 92:570 (Letter).
70. Swanson, M. A., Chanmougan, D., and Schwartz, R. S. (1966): Immunohemolytic anemia due to antipenicillin antibodies. *N. Engl. J. Med.*, 274:178–181.
71. Takahara, S. (1968): Acatalasemia in Japan. In: *Hereditary Disorders of Erythrocyte Metabolism* edited by E. Beutler, pp. 21–40. City of Hope Symposium Series, Vol. I, Grune & Stratton, New York.
72. Thomson, C. D., Rea, H. M., Doesburg, V. M., and Robinson, M. F. (1977): Selenium concentrations and glutathione peroxidase activities in whole blood of New Zealand residents. *Br. J. Nutr.*, 37:457–460.
73. Tschirren, B. (1983): Phenazopyridine-induced hemolytic anemia in a patient with G-6-PD deficiency. *Acta Haematol.*, 70:208–209.
74. Valentine, W. N., Paglia, D. E., Fink, K., and Madokoro, G. (1976): Lead poisoning. Association with hemolytic anemia, basophilic stippling, erythrocyte pyrimidine 5'-nucleotidase deficiency, and intraerythrocytic accumulation of pyrimidines. *J. Clin. Invest.*, 58:926–932.
75. Van Arsdel, P. P. Jr., and Gilliland, B. C. (1965): Anemia secondary to penicillin treatment: Studies on two patients with non-allergic serum hemagglutinins. *J. Lab. Clin. Med.*, 65:277–285.
76. Waldron, H. A. (1966): The anaemia of lead poisoning: A review. *Br. J. Ind. Med.*, 23:83–100.
77. Wenz, B., Klein, R. L., and Lalezari, P. (1974): Tetracycline-induced immune hemolytic anemia. *Transfusion*, 14:265–269.
78. Westerman, M. P., Pfitzer, E., Ellis, L. D., and Jensen, W. N. (1965): Concentrations of lead in bone in plumbism. *N. Engl. J. Med.*, 273:1246–1250.
79. White, J. M., Brown, D. L., Hepner, G. W., and Worlledge, S. M. (1968): Penicillin induced hemolytic anaemia. *Br. Med. J.*, 3:26–29.
80. Woolley, P. V. III, Sacher, R. A., Priego, V. M., Schanfield, M. S., and Bonnem, E. M. (1983): Methotrexate-induced immune haemolytic anaemia. *Br. J. Haematol.*, 54:543–552.
81. Yano, S., Danish, E. and Hsia, Y. E. (1982): Transient methemoglobinemia with acidosis in infants. *J. Pediatr.*, 100:415–418.

Toxicology of the Blood and Bone Marrow,
edited by Richard D. Irons. Raven Press,
New York © 1985.

Chemical Toxicity of the Granulocyte

John C. Marsh

Yale University School of Medicine, New Haven, Connecticut 06510

The influence of chemical agents on circulating blood granulocytes may be divided into (a) effects on the function of the mature cell and (b) effects on the number of circulating cells in the blood. In turn, cell number may be considered from the standpoint of decreased production by the marrow, increased destruction, or changes in the ratio of circulating cells, which are counted, and marginated cells, which are not.

In this chapter consideration is limited to neutrophilic granulocytes, not only because they are more numerous than eosinophilic and basophilic granulocytes, but because much more information is available about their function, regulation of production, and kinetics.

Neutrophils normally leave the bone marrow as mature cells, with a complement of both primary (azurophilic) and secondary (specific neutrophilic) granules, which are full of various enzymes that perform specific tasks. Mature cells are recognized as such in the blood as either mature polymorphonuclear (PMN) cells or as slightly less mature band forms. They enter the blood and remain in it with a half-life of about 7 hours and leave it randomly, passing between capillary endothelial cells into the tissues where they perform their major task, that of being the advance guard of phagocytes against invading microorganisms. Clearly, anything that interferes with either the normal function of these cells or their number can predispose the host to infection, which may be lethal.

NEUTROPHIL FUNCTION

In considering neutrophil function (14), it is important to distinguish between studies *in vitro*, in which a drug or chemical is added in varying concentration to isolated normal cells whose function is then measured, and *in vivo* studies, in which PMNs are removed from animals or patients who have been given the drug under study and whose function is then compared with that of normal cells. The latter type of study is more meaningful but, unfortunately, information of this type is not always available.

What does a mature PMN do? Neutrophil function can be broadly subdivided into the migration cascade, or sequence, and the killing cascade. The former includes the processes of margination, adherence and aggregation, diapedesis through

51

the vessel wall, and migration directed through a chemotactic stimulus. The killing cascade includes recognition, attachment, phagocytosis, granule fusion, degranulation and respiratory burst associated with intracellular killing, digestion and exocytosis of microorganisms.

By adherence is meant the attachment of cells to vascular endothelium prior to their leaving the blood to passage between these same endothelial cells. The complex changes occurring in diabetes, as well as in the presence of ethanol, have been reported to inhibit this process. Epinephrine can cause a very rapid increase in the concentration of PMNs in the circulating blood by demargination, presumably also by interfering with PMN adherence. Histamine, iron oxide, and dextran, on the other hand, appear to enhance the process of margination, causing a "pseudoneutropenia." Colchicine inhibits the adherence process, presumably through its effect on microtubules, which are required, along with microfilaments, for normal adherence.

Chemotaxis means the directed movement of cells in response to a concentration gradient of a mediator. Among the known chemotactic factors are bacterial components, those derived from the complement system, those derived from Hageman factor activation, and those derived from the PMN itself, including cyclic AMP and certain prostaglandins. Endotoxin, cellular necrosis, antigen-antibody complexes, and nonspecific tissue damage may attract neutrophils by various combinations of these mechanisms.

The process of chemotaxis is most commonly studied *in vitro*, using a chamber in which the cells to be studied are separated from the chemotactic stimulus by a filter that can then be examined for the extent of PMN migration through it (6). Its *in vivo* counterpart is the skin window (21) in which coverslips are placed over a skin abrasion, with or without a bacterial stimulus, and examined quantitatively over time for the rate of appearance of PMNs.

Microtubules within the cell are important in the chemotactic process. The function of these structures is inhibited by colchicine, vincristine, and vinblastine, as well as by halothane. Colchicine, as well as actinomycin D, has also been reported to interfere with the elaboration of a chemotactic factor produced by PMNs after they ingest urate crystals.

The PMNs of colchicine-treated patients, however, have been reported to have normal chemotactic responses *in vitro*, but a decreased response to inflammatory skin windows. Increased levels of cyclic AMP inhibit chemotaxis, and the action of histamine, various β-adrenergic agents, theophylline, and certain prostaglandins has been explained in this way. On the other hand, increased levels of cyclic GMP enhance chemotaxis, and various cholinergic drugs, as well as levamisole, are thought to act in this fashion. High doses of vitamin C also enhance chemotaxis.

Several anti-inflammatory agents are *in vitro* inhibitors of chemotaxis. These include hydrocortisone, methyl prednisolone, chloroquine, quinine, and phenylbutazone, whereas aspirin is without effect. The relatively high concentrations that were needed to show this effect, however, raise some question about the significance of the observation. The intravenous (i.v.) injection of a large dose of hydrocortisone, however, did inhibit the accumulation of PMNs at skin windows as well as cause an increase in the rate of marrow input of PMNs into the blood (2).

Other inhibitors of chemotaxis, based on *in vitro* studies, include the antibiotics tetracycline, rifampin, chloramphenicol, and amphotericin B. Also identified as inhibitors are chlorpromazine, penicillamine, ethanol, heparin, and caffeine.

Phagocytosis is the engulfment of a particle and its sequestration in an intracellular vacuole. One can measure the rate of uptake of particles over a period of time or the number of particles per cell at a specific time. The percentage of cells that contains ingested particles can also be measured. The phagocytic process is also inhibited by cyclic AMP and enhanced by increased intracellular levels of cyclic GMP and therefore is influenced by the same agents that affect these cyclic nucleotides, as mentioned above under chemotaxis. Elevated levels of the sugars galactose and glucose inhibit phagocytosis, thus providing a suggestive explanation for the increased susceptibility to infection seen in galactosemia as well as the much more common diabetes mellitus. Colchicine has been reported both to inhibit and to have no effect on phagocytosis.

Degranulation is the delivery of the granule contents of the PMN into the phagocytic vacuole or into the extracellular environment. Intracellular degranulation is inhibited by colchicine and vinblastine through their effects on microtubules, and by theophylline, histamine, and β-adrenergic agents. The process is enhanced by cholinergic agents. Degranulation into the extracellular environment is inhibited by corticosteroids and chloroquine.

Phagocytosis or, indeed, even perturbation of the plasma membrane of the cell triggers a burst of oxygen consumption, increased glucose utilization, including activation of the hexose monophosphate shunt, generation of a superoxide anion, which is important in intracellular killing, and chemiluminescence. Colchicine and vinblastine have been reported to interfere with the generation of superoxide anion.

The antimicrobial systems in the PMN are those that are oxygen dependent, including that mediated by myeloperoxidase and that inhibited by various sulfonamides and antithyroid agents, and oxygen-independent systems, which include killing mediated by lysozyme, lactoferrin, and various cationic proteins found in the granules.

Lithium carbonate has well-defined stimulatory effects on leukocyte production and is being used to protect against the neutropenia produced by various antineoplastic agents. When the PMNs of normal volunteers were studied before and after the ingestion of lithium, they were found to have normal mobilization to skin windows, nitroblue tetrazolium reduction (as a measure of superoxide anion production), normal chemotaxis in a Boyden chamber to bacterial products, normal phagocytosis, and chemiluminescence but impaired intracellular killing of ingested *Staphylococcus aureus* (10). The importance of this observation relative to the beneficial effect of lithium on neutrophil production remains to be determined.

Ethanol has multiple inhibitory effects on PMN: not only is there impaired production, but there is diminished cellular adherence, decreased chemotaxis *in vitro* (although skin window tests of acutely intoxicated patients are normal), and diminished phagocytosis. Diabetes has been associated with decreased PMN adherence, chemotaxis, phagocytosis, and intracellular killing. Among the defects described in chronic renal failure and in the resulting symptom complex known as uremia is impaired chemotaxis, but phagocytosis and intracellular killing of organisms have been found to be normal in most studies.

REDUCED NEUTROPHIL NUMBERS (NEUTROPENIA)

In theory, a reduction in the number of circulating granulocytes in the blood (9) may come about by inadequate production in the marrow, excessive peripheral destruction or utilization, or by a shift of the circulating granulocytes into the blood marginal pool, a situation that has been referred to as "pseudoneutropenia." Inadequate production of neutrophils is by far the most common effect of pharmacologic agents. Reduced granulocytopoiesis may be predictable or unpredictable (idiosyncratic).

Predictable neutropenia is the type seen commonly with cancer chemotherapeutic agents, which do not distinguish between normal and cancer cells. It develops slowly and is dose dependent. It may rise from direct stem cell damage, from interruption of DNA synthesis, the binding or depolymerization of DNA, inhibition of mitosis, or interference with protein synthesis. Examples, in addition to most antineoplastic agents, are chloramphenicol, rifampin, ristocetin, benzene, ethanol, and nitrous oxide. We return to a more detailed consideration of this type of toxicity, particularly with respect to stem cells, in the discussion below.

Idiosyncratic drug-induced interference with granulopoiesis may be of two types: that which is slow to develop and dose dependent and that which appears to be a hypersensitivity reaction and occurs rapidly. In the former, certain types of people are at increased risk: the old more than the young, female more than male, and white more than black. It is thought to be an individual sensitivity of DNA and RNA synthesis, at least with the prototype, which is chlorpromazine intoxication. The onset is usually between 2 and 3 weeks after drug ingestion, and the incidence is of the order of 1 in 1,000 to 2,000. Among the drugs implicated in this type of delayed idiosyncratic inhibition of granulocyte production are phenothiazines, chloramphenicol, acetaminophen (Tylenol), carbenicillin, butazolidine, propylthiouracil, sulfa drugs, and procaine amide.

The rare idiosyncratic neutropenia that appears to be a hypersensitivity reaction develops within a few days of beginning drug ingestion. It is usually associated with prior ingestion of the drug and with eosinophilia. Recovery is usually prompt, but may be slow. Drugs causing it often contain a benzene ring; they include chloramphenicol, gold salts, phenylbutazone, sulfas, isoniazid, indomethacin, procaine amide, ampicillin, nitrofurantoin, propylthiouracil, and chlorothiazide.

Several drugs are associated with what seems to be ineffective granulopoiesis, that is, an intramedullary death of granulocyte precursors. This is the picture seen with vitamin B_{12} or folate deficiency and that has been described with diphenylhydantoin, pyrimethamine, ethanol, and chloramphenicol. This type of neutropenia develops slowly and is often dose dependent and predictable.

Turning to increased granulocyte destruction, the neutrophil analog of hemolytic anemia, some drugs cause an immune destruction of granulocytes mediated through an antibody. This may happen within hours if the patient has been previously exposed to the drug and within a few days after initial exposure. The classic drug so implicated is aminopyrine; serum from a sensitized patient and the drug together will produce neutropenia in a normal patient, but neither is sufficient when given alone. Rarely, phenylbutazone and sulfa drugs produce neutropenia through a similar mechanism. Antibodies that agglutinate neutrophils *in vitro* have been found in some patients with neutropenia and with a history of ingesting the following drugs: gold salts, chloroquine, barbiturates, methyldopa, and phenothiazines. The exact significance of these agglutinins in producing neutropenia is uncertain.

Redistribution neutropenia, or "pseudoneutropenia," is an increase in the marginal granulocyte pool at the expense of the circulating pool, but with no net change in the total blood granulocyte pool. Histamine, dextran, and iron oxide have all been reported to effect this redistribution.

Myelosuppression is the most common side effect of cancer chemotherapy, except for nausea and vomiting, and is responsible for more serious disability, time spent in hospital, and deaths than any other toxicity from this cause. Although red cell production may be more sensitive than white cell or platelet production to most drugs (3), the long intravascular life-span of red cells compared with white cells and platelets, coupled with the availability of red cells for transfusion, makes the anemia resulting from chemotherapy a relatively minor problem. The longer life-span of platelets in blood compared with neutrophils and *their* availability for transfusion makes thrombocytopenia less serious than neutropenia.

Most combination chemotherapy regimens contain at least two agents with the potential for marrow toxicity: failure to decrease the dose of these agents compared with their maximal tolerated dose when given as single agents can produce unacceptable toxicity. Reducing the dose, however, can compromise the antitumor efficacy of the regimen, which may explain the lack of advantage of many combinations compared with single agents.

Myelosuppression is so ubiquitous that drugs that don't cause it are unusual and make favorite ingredients for combination regimens, at times even when their intrinsic activity against a particular tumor is low. Bleomycin in small-cell cancer of the lung regimens is an example. Drugs with little or no potential for myelosuppression include the steroid hormones (glucocorticosteroids, androgens, estrogens, progestins, antiestrogens), L-asparaginase, o,p'DDD(mitotane), and spirogermanium. Vincristine, bleomycin, and streptozotocin cause little myelosuppression when used in patients with normal marrows and good liver function, but the potential for myelosuppression is there in compromised patients. Dacarbazine (DTIC) and cisplatin produce relatively mild marrow toxicity because other toxicities are dose-limiting.

What factors determine drug toxicity for the bone marrow? They include host factors such as age, nutritional status, hepatic and renal function, involvement of the marrow by tumor, prior therapy including both radiotherapy and chemotherapy, the proliferative state of the marrow, and the presence or absence of infection, particularly with endotoxin-producing organisms. Drug-related factors include the dose, route of administration, schedule, mechanism of action, pharmacokinetics, and sensitivity of specific target cells within the marrow.

Older patients tolerate chemotherapeutic agents less well than younger patients, presumably because of a decreased cellularity, i.e., a smaller total marrow mass (13). Likewise, patients with poor nutritional status, evidenced by weight loss, have a diminished tolerance for chemotherapy and greater myelosuppression (8).

Organ function can play a major role in determining any type of toxicity, including myelosuppression. The liver is important in the metabolism and excretion of such drugs as doxorubicin (Adriamycin) and the other anthracyclines, 5-fluorouracil (5-FU), cytosine arabinoside, the vinca alkaloids, and mitomycin C; failure to reduce the dose of these agents in patients with impaired liver function may result in lethal myelosuppression. Cyclophosphamide (CY) is *activated* by the liver and may be less effective (or myelotoxic) in the presence of impaired liver function. Similarly, impaired renal function may prolong the effect of certain agents, producing severe toxicity. This is most noteworthy for methotrexate, which is excreted almost entirely by the kidney. Cisplatin is also heavily dependent on renal excretion and has the potential for causing substantial additional renal toxicity and myelosuppression if given to a patient with reduced renal function.

Failure to consider the state of the bone marrow can lead to major problems. If the marrow is infiltrated by tumor, peripheral blood counts may be normal or low, with varying qualitative changes characteristic of myelophthisic anemia. Although treatment with chemotherapy can be hazardous, it may in fact be appropriate to be aggressive, as improvement cannot occur without killing tumor cells. On the other hand, if the marrow is severely compromised by the effects of prior irradiation or chemotherapy, no amount of tumor-cell killing is likely to help, and the dose must be reduced to avoid fatal results. Bone marrow aspiration and biopsy will be helpful. It should be remembered that a compromised marrow may still maintain normal peripheral blood counts. Tests of marrow granulocyte reserve with etiocholanolone, endotoxin, or prednisone are available. The integrity of the marrow may be presumed to be compromised if neutropenia develops earlier than a week after administration of a myelotoxic agent, since a normal marrow granulocyte storage pool should be able to maintain a normal circulating neutrophil level for that time. A marrow struggling to maintain a normal neutrophil count will release young cells into the blood; thus, the neutrophil band:seg ratio may be increased and suggest marrow impairment or incomplete recovery from prior therapy. It is important to realize that for both phase-specific and cycle-specific agents, rapidly proliferating marrow precursors (stem cells and more differentiated, morphologically recognizable progeny) are more sensitive to drugs than the cells of a resting marrow.

The importance of considering the proliferative state of the bone marrow is shown by the fact that a specific dose of CY may be well tolerated initially without significant leukopenia, but a second, identical dose given 12 days later produces a sharp fall in the level of blood neutrophils. This can be explained by increased sensitivity of the neutrophil precursors, which are rapidly proliferating to recover from the cytotoxicity and cell kill caused by the first dose.

The presence of endotoxin-producing organisms may be important in determining host tolerance to chemotherapy. Not only may the marrow be proliferating in response to the infection, and therefore be more drug sensitive, but pharmacokinetics may be influenced by endotoxins. Changes in plasma clearance, volume of distribution, and urinary excretion of several anticancer agents have been produced by endotoxin in experimental animals (15). The effect on the concentration × time ($C \times t$) product can be either increased or decreased, depending on the agent. It was suggested that endotoxin may also affect the drug penetration of various organs.

The dose of the drug is the most obvious variable that can affect the magnitude of neutropenia. As doses of CY, for example, are increased in groups of patients, the magnitude of peripheral blood neutropenia and its duration increases. Most agents with myelosuppressive potential, except S-phase specific drugs such as methotrexate and cytosine arabinoside (19), exhibit an exponential dose-response curve for stem cells that are committed to neutrophil-macrophage colony formation (16,18). The phase-specific agents produce plateau dose-response curves. Such curves, generally measuring the effect early after drug administration, can be helpful in comparing the effect of different drugs on the same species, or the same drug in different species, but a full understanding requires stem cell recovery curves, generally available only in the mouse (5).

The importance of the route of administration is shown by the fact that doxorubicin, 5-FU, or 5-fluorodeoxyuridine can be given directly into the liver where they are metabolized via the hepatic artery in doses that would be prohibitively toxic if given intravenously. Optimal doses for specific routes of administration must be derived from phase I trials.

The importance of schedule is shown by the experience with cytosine arabinoside. When the time of continuous infusion of a specific dose was lengthened from 24 to 48 to 96 hours in solid-tumor patients, the degree and duration of neutropenia were progressively increased. The increase is the result of a larger number of neutrophil precursors in the bone marrow coming into contact with this DNA synthesis (S)-phase specific agent during the longer time period.

Drugs that are myelotoxic have varying degrees of myelosuppression time to nadir and time to recovery (13). Drugs with the shortest times to nadir include the vinca alkaloids; slightly longer times are seen with the anthracyclines, alkylating agents, and antimetabolites; long times to nadir and recovery are seen with the nitrosoureas, busulfan, mitomycin, and procarbazine (Table 1). With the latter agents it appears as if there is incomplete recovery in many patients. A predominant action on early marrow precursors seems likely. The kinetics of recovery and a relatively selective effect on different precursor cells by different drugs have been demonstrated by Botnick et al. (5). They compared the effect of several agents on (a) mouse marrow CFU-S (colony-forming unit, spleen), a multipotent stem cell capable of red cell, granulocyte-macrophage, and megakaryocyte differentiation

TABLE 1. *Comparison of neutrophil nadir and recovery*
for four anticancer agents

	Nadir (days)	Recovery (days)
X-ray "mantle"	14	90
Alkylating agent (nitrogen mustard)	10	21
Antimetabolite (cytosine arabinoside)	14	28
Nitrosourea (Lomustine, CCNU)	35–42	50–60

and (b) the ADCPC (agar diffusion chamber precursor cell), a stem cell committed to granulocyte-macrophage production. The self-renewal capacity for CFU-S was also measured. ADCPCs were more sensitive than CFU-S at 24 hours to velban, equally sensitive to 5-FU and CY, and were *less* sensitive than CFU-S to carmustine (BCNU) and busulfan. Bone marrow CFU-S recovery curves showed a later nadir and recovery after BCNU and busulfan than after CY and 5-FU. Of most interest was the failure of the self-renewal capacity of CFU-S to return to normal after BCNU and busulfan, compared with 5-FU and CY, even after 5 months. Recovery after BCNU was not even seen after 22 months. Clearly, different drugs are able to influence important marrow precursor cells at different points in their proliferation and maturation pathway.

Since 1975 we have used the ADCPC assay to compare the effects of different anticancer drugs on bone marrow granulocyte-macrophage stem cells from different species. The assay can also be used to measure drug effects on tumor stem cells as well. The ADC technique (11) has two advantages over *in vitro* assays: (a) It does not require a source of purified, stable, colony-stimulating factor; (b) the drug(s) to be tested can be injected directly into the chamber-bearing mouse and thus undergo *in vivo* activation, distribution, metabolism, and excretion as it interacts with the bone marrow clonogenic cells (12).

We have done two types of assay: dose-response experiments in which the bone marrow is exposed to the drug *in situ* (only in the mouse) and then assayed for surviving colony-forming cells; and dose-response experiments in which mouse, human, or canine marrow is exposed to the drug while it is suspended in the ADC. The drug is given i.v. and after a fixed time (usually 18 hours) the chamber is transplanted into a normal mouse for incubation of 7 to 14 days, depending on the marrow species. Thus, the sensitivity of mouse marrow in the chamber can be compared with that *in situ* and also with marrow from dog and man. Correlations with toxicology studies in animals and phase I clinical trials were made. It should be possible to predict the potential for the production of neutropenia by a new drug in humans without ever exposing patients to it.

As described by Bruce et al. (7), two types of dose-response curve are seen. The first type is exponential, reflecting first-order kinetics of clonogenic cell kill

(Fig. 1). This means that the population of colony-forming cells is killed in a fixed proportion for each increment of a drug over the range studied and that the dose-survival curve is a straight line when plotted on semilogarithmic paper. Doses that produce a specific cell survival (D_{37} = dose that kills 63% of the cells) can be calculated and these doses compared for different species. When we studied dox-orubicin, we found similar sensitivities for mouse marrow *in situ*, and in the chamber, and for human marrow (D_{37} values of 8,8, and 9 mg/kg), but dog marrow was much more sensitive (3.5 mg/kg) (18). From toxicologic studies the dog is known to be the most sensitive of these species to the drug, whose limiting toxicity is granulocytopenia. The anthracycline derivative, AD-32, has a similar order of marrow sensitivity, although human cells are relatively more sensitive than to doxorubicin. It was predicted that granulocytopenia would be the limiting human toxicity for AD-32 also; such, indeed, is the case (4). Carminomycin, a Russian drug, and aclacinomycin A from Japan, other anthracycline derivatives, also have exponential dose-response curves. Marcellomycin, with little white cell toxicity in mice, has a flat mouse marrow *in situ* curve, but a steep exponential one for human

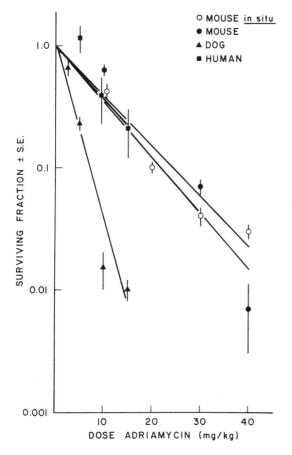

FIG. 1. Dose-survival curves of bone marrow agar diffusion chamber precursor cells from different species 18 hours after adriamycin. (With permission from Marsh, ref. 18.)

marrow. Recent clinical studies with marcellomycin have shown granulocytopenia to be dose limiting. A new agent, dibenzyldaunomycin, has exponential curves for the three species; it may be predicted to have a leukopenia-producing single dose in man of approximately 200 mg/m^2.

When five anthracyclines that we have tested are ranked for their potency against human marrow in the assay and compared with the single dose producing a given level of neutropenia in man, the agreement is excellent (Table 2) (20). Other drugs with exponential dose-survival curves in the ADCPC assay include CY, 5-FU, cisplatin, DTIC, methyl-GAG, amsacrine (m-AMSA), mitomycin C, and pyrazafurin. There are, however, definite differences in the slopes of the curves for different species, and the species sensitivities vary from drug to drug; they are not predictable (17).

The other type of dose-survival curve is a plateau in which only a limited number of colony-forming cells are killed, regardless of the dose of drug given (Fig. 2). This is because the drug kills cells only in a certain phase of the cell cycle, and, in some instances because of the ability of the drug to cause a delay or block in passage through the cycle.

The location of the plateau is determined also by the pharmacokinetics of the drug; i.e., how long the population is exposed to a cytotoxic concentration of drug. Since this is the same when the marrows from different species are exposed to the drug in the chamber, a true picture of comparative species sensitivities can be obtained. Drugs that produce plateau dose-survival curves include the antifolates methotrexate, triazinate (Baker's antifol), JB-11, a trimethoxyquinazoline derivative about to enter clinical trial, cytosine arabinoside (19), and 5-azacytidine. Estramustine produces a plateau for dog and human ADCPC but an exponential curve for mouse marrow cells. Differences in species sensitivity are usually slight, but again, not consistent or predictable.

Spirogermanium, a drug without any *in vivo* myelosuppressive effect against mice, dogs, or humans, has no effect on colony formation in the ADC assay.

The effect of two-drug combinations can also be tested in this system. A combination of methotrexate and 5-FU is of current clinical interest and appears to be synergistic in killing some kinds of tumors. Naturally, the therapeutic index

TABLE 2. *Comparison of D$_{37}$ dose for human marrow and single i.v. leukopenia-producing dose in phase I and II studies*

Drug	D$_{37}$ (mg/m^2)	Leukopenia-producing dose (mg/m^2)	Median WBC
Carminomycin	3.3	20	2.9
Marcellomycin	13.5	40	3.0
Aclacinomycin A	18.0	100	3.0
Adriamycin	38.5	60–75	3.0
AD$_{32}$	66.0	400	3.2

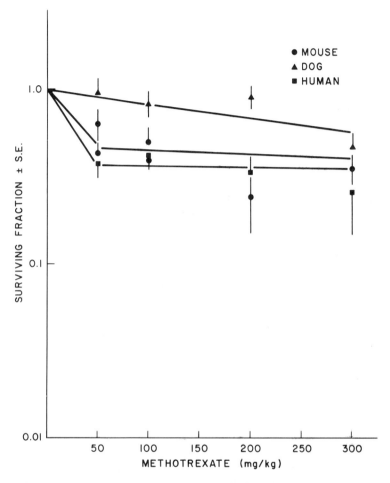

FIG. 2. Dose-survival curves of bone marrow agar diffusion chamber precursor cells from different species 18 hours after methotrexate. (With permission from Marsh, ref. 19.)

depends on whether or not this combination also kills marrow colony-forming cells synergistically as well. Some preliminary data with marrow from all three species suggest that it does not. Likewise, it has been shown that pretreatment of mice with allopurinol will protect them from 5-FU lethality (24). We have observed that allopurinol protects marrow ADCPC in mice from this drug, which may explain at least part of this effect (23).

After chemotherapy, during the marrow recovery phase, the concentration of white cell colony-forming cells in the blood, where they are normally present in low concentration, may be markedly increased (1,22). Such an expansion of circulating colony-forming cells in the blood may potentially be of value in reconstituting patients following high-dose chemotherapy or irradiation.

In conclusion, the leukocyte-committed colony-forming cell (ADCPC or CFU-culture) is probably the most relevant population for the study of hematological toxicity in man, since leukopenia is the most potentially lethal complication of such toxicity. It can be studied serially over a period of time in the blood or marrow, as well as evaluated for sensitivity to specific drugs in specific individuals. The assay is potentially of value in predicting the likelihood that a given drug will produce significant neutropenia in man without the necessity for clinical trial. In combination with assays of tumor stem cell drug sensitivity, it may be possible to design optimal chemotherapy for cancer patients in a much more rational fashion than hitherto has been the case.

ACKNOWLEDGMENTS

This work was supported by grant Ch-37 from the American Cancer Society and grants CA 18341 and CA 08341 from the National Cancer Institute.

REFERENCES

1. Abrams, R. A., McCormack, K., Bowles, C., and Deisseroth, A. B. (1981): Cyclophosphamide treatment expands the circulating hematopoietic stem cell pool in dogs. *J. Clin. Invest.*, 67:1392–1399.
2. Bishop, C. R., Athens, J. W., Boggs, D. R., Warner, H. R., Cartwright, G. E., and Wintrobe, M. M. (1968): Leukokinetic Studies. XIII. A nonsteady state kinetic evaluation of the mechanism of cortisone-induced granulocytosis. *J. Clin. Invest.*, 50:920–930.
3. Blackett, N. M., Marsh, J. C., Gordon, M. Y., Okell, S. F., and Aguado, M. (1978): The simultaneous assay by six methods of the effect on haemopoietic precursor cells of adriamycin, methyl-CCNU, β-rays, vinblastine and cytosine arabinoside. *Exp. Hematol.*, 6:2–8.
4. Blum, R. H., Henderson, I. C., Mayer, R. J., Skarin, A. T., Parker, L. M., Canellos, G. P., Israel, M., and Frei, E., III. (1979): Phase I—evaluation of N-trifluoroacetyladriamycin-14-valerate (AD-32) and adriamycin (A) analog. *Proc. Am. Soc. Clin. Oncol. Am. Assoc. Cancer Res.*, 20:327.
5. Botnick, L. E., Hannon, E. C., Vigneulle, R., and Hellman, S. (1981): Differential effects of cytotoxic agents on hematopoietic progenitors. *Cancer Res.*, 41:2338–2342.
6. Boyden, S. (1962): The chemotactic effect of mixtures of antibody and antigen on polymorphonuclear leukocytes. *J. Exp. Med.*, 115:453–466.
7. Bruce, W. R., Meeker, B. E., and Valeriote, F. A. (1966): Comparison of the sensitivity of normal hematopoietic and transplanted lymphoma colony-forming cells to chemotherapeutic agents administered *in vivo*. *J. Natl. Cancer Inst.*, 37:233–245.
8. Dewys, W. D., Begg, C., and Lavin, P. T. (1980): Prognostic effect of weight loss prior to chemotherapy in cancer patients. *Am. J. Med.*, 69:491–497.
9. Finch, S. C. (1977): Granulocytopenia. In: *Hematology*, edited by W. J. Williams, E. Beutler, A. J. Ersley, and R. W. Rundles, pp. 717–746. McGraw-Hill, New York, 2nd ed.
10. Friedenberg, W. R., and Marx, J. J., Jr. (1980): The effect of lithium carbonate on lymphocyte, granulocyte and platelet function. *Cancer*, 45:91–97.
11. Gordon, M. Y. (1974): Quantitation of haemopoietic cells from normal and leukaemic RFM mice using an *in vivo* colony assay. *Br. J. Cancer*, 30:421–428.
12. Gordon, M. Y., and Blackett, N. M. (1976): The sensitivities of human and murine hemopoietic cells exposed to cytotoxic drugs in an *in vivo* culture system. *Cancer Res.*, 36:2822–2826.
13. Hoagland, H. C. (1982): Hematologic complications of cancer chemotherapy. *Semin. Oncol.*, 9:95–102.
14. Klebanoff, S. J., and Clark, R. A. (1978): *The Neutrophil: Function and Disorders*. North Holland Publishing Co., Amsterdam-New York-Oxford.
15. Lu, K., Rosenblum, M. G., and Loo, T. L. (1981): Effects of endotoxin on the pharmacology of antineoplastic agents. *Cancer Chemother. Pharmacol.*, 5:277–231.

16. Marsh, J. C. (1976): The effects of cancer chemotherapeutic agents on normal hematopoietic precursor cells: A review. *Cancer Res.*, 36:1853–1882.
17. Marsh, J. C. (1978): The comparative sensitivity of marrow colony-forming cells to anticancer drugs: canine, human and mouse studies. *Exp. Hematol.*, [6, *Suppl.*] 3:79.
18. Marsh, J. C. (1979): A comparison of the sensitivities of human, canine and murine hematopoietic precursor cells to adriamycin and N-tri-fluoroacetyladriamycin-14-valerate. *Cancer Res.*, 39:360–364.
19. Marsh, J. C. (1982): Comparative effects of methotrexate, two nonclassical folic acid antagonists, and cytarabine on hematopoietic precursor cells. *Cancer Treat. Rep.*, 66:499–504.
20. Marsh, J. C., Brown, B. J., and Nierenburg, M. (1983): Sensitivity of bone marrow hematopoietic colony-forming cells from mice, dog and humans to carminomycin, marcellomycin, aclacinomycin A and N,N-dibenzyldaunorubicin, and its relationship to clinical toxicity. *Cancer Res.*, 43:2962–2966.
21. Rebuck, J. W., and Crowley, J. H. (1955): A method of studying leukocytic function *in vivo. Ann. NY Acad. Sci.*, 59:757–794.
22. Richman, C. M., Weiner, R. S., and Yankee, R. A. (1976): Increase in circulating stem cells following chemotherapy in man. *Blood*, 47:1031–1039.
23. Schwartz, P. M., Dunigan, J. M., Marsh, J. C., and Handschumacher, R. E. (1980): Allopurinol modification of the toxicity and antitumor activity of 5-fluorouracil. *Cancer Res.*, 40:1885–1889.
24. Schwartz, P. M., and Handschumacher, R. E. (1979): Selective antagonism of 5-fluorouracil cytotoxicity by 4-hydroxypyrazolopyrimidine (allopurinol) *in vitro. Cancer Res.*, 39:3095–3101.

Toxicology of the Blood and Bone Marrow,
edited by Richard D. Irons. Raven Press,
New York © 1985.

Clonogenic Stem and Progenitor Cell Assays for the Evaluation of Chemically Induced Myelotoxicity

Floyd D. Wilson

*U.S. Department of Agriculture, Western Regional Research Center,
Albany, California 94710*

The hemopoietic and immune systems contain cellular targets that are uniquely sensitive to a wide variety of toxic physical and chemical agents. The cellular components of these systems are members of an elaborate cell renewal system in which constant cellular proliferation must be maintained to meet the demand imposed by loss of the mature effector cell products. Thus, lymphohemopoietic elements are particularly responsive to chemical agents with radiomimetic properties.

The development of methods to assay for the adverse effects of chemical agents on hemopoietic stem and progenitor cells is of major importance to the field of toxicology. In addition to the direct relevancy to myelotoxicity, studies on hemopoiesis also provide a unique model for the investigation of cell regulation and for the examination of basic pathogenetic mechanisms associated with toxicity. This, in part, is due to the relatively "fluid" nature of hemopoietic tissues which facilitates isolation of the individual cellular components. Isolation of single cells cannot be readily achieved for "solid" tissue systems. Thus, individual cells can be isolated, independently characterized, and reintroduced into culture under controlled conditions facilitating studies on mechanisms involved in cellular regulation, amplification, and differentiation.

In this chapter, methods for the study of toxic effects produced on the stem and progenitor cells for lymphohemopoiesis are reviewed, emphasizing techniques that allow for the *in vitro* clonal growth of the various classes of lymphohemopoietic progenitor cells (1) and the application of such techniques to investigations on myelotoxicity.

REVIEW OF NORMAL HEMOPOIESIS

The study of mechanisms involved in myelotoxicity requires a basic understanding of the fundamental components involved in the regulation of lymphohemopoiesis (2). One model for hemopoiesis (Fig. 1) suggests the presence of populations of

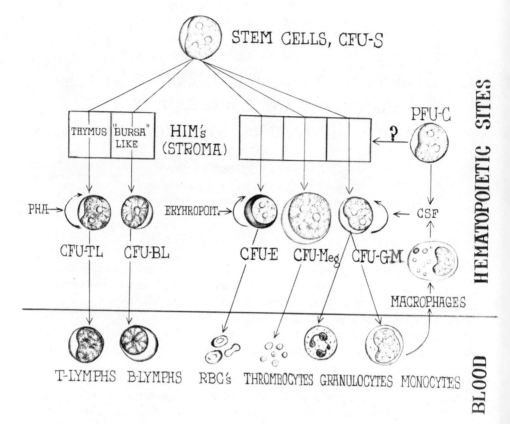

FIG. 1. Current concepts of lymphohemopoiesis. CFU-S, colony-forming units; spleen, pluripotent stem cells; HIM, hemopoietic stromal microenvironments; PFU-C, fibroblast colony-forming unit; CFU-TL, colony-forming unit for T lymphocytes; CFU-BL, colony-forming unit for B lymphocytes; CFU-E, colony-forming unit for erythrocytes; CFU-Meg, colony-forming unit for megakaryocytes; CFU-C, colony-forming unit for granulocytes and monocyte/macrophages; CSF, colony-stimulating factor, "granulopoietin"; PHA, phytohemagglutinin.

pluripotent hemopoietic stem cells (colony-forming units in spleen, CFU-S), "stromal-associated" hemopoietic and lymphopoietic microenvironments, populations of "committed" stem or progenitor cells, and various humoral regulators (hormones or poietins) that are thought to exert their influence primarily at the level of the committed progenitor cells. The fundamental components of the model include a capacity for self-renewal, amplification, and pluripotent stem cell differentiation.

It is important to recognize that although the model for hemopoiesis (Fig. 1) depicts the various stages of differentiation as being discreet compartments or steps, hemopoietic development undoubtedly is a gradual and continuous differentiation process. Thus, numerous successive stages of cells with various degrees of replicative and differentiative capacities undoubtedly exist. In general, the capacity for self-renewal and proliferation is inversely related to the differentiation state. In addition, many components of the model remain hypothetical and controversial.

The lymphohemopoietic system in adult mammals is relatively unique by virtue of its extensive capacity for cell renewal. Since the mature cells of this system are consistently consumed through senescence or removed from the body, a finely regulated mechanism to balance cell production with cell loss is necessary for the maintenance of hemopoiesis. In addition, mechanisms must exist for rapid expansion of lymphohemopoietic elements in response to the many recurrent pathological insults to the body.

Any system in which embryonic demands for cellular proliferation persist throughout adulthood requires a pool of stem cells, which, by definition, must exhibit the property of self-renewal to maintain their own kind. In addition, stem cells must maintain a supply of a wide variety of morphologically and functionally diverse lymphohemopoietic elements; that process requires a pluripotent differentiation capacity. Thus, populations of stem cells capable of both self-renewal and pluripotent cellular differentiation must be maintained throughout the life of an animal. These are the pluripotent hemopoietic stem cells (3), which were described previously in the chapter by E. Cronkite, *this volume*.

In addition to the self-replicating pluripotent hemopoietic stem cells, populations of partially differentiated progenitor cells have also been identified. Such partially differentiated progenitors, although maintaining the capacity for proliferation, are no longer pluripotent but, rather, have differentiation capacities restricted to a single pathway of lymphohemopoiesis and thus are termed committed stem or progenitor cells.

Regulators of hemopoiesis can be divided into two major groups: humoral regulators (hormones or poietins) and cellular regulators, including possible "stromal-based" microenvironmental influences. A wide variety of specific humoral regulators of hemopoiesis have been identified (Fig. 1). Growth and differentiation factors have been shown to exert their major effects at the level of the committed progenitor cells (1), although humoral regulators of pluripotent stem cells have recently been described (4). The best characterized humoral regulator is erythropoietin (Epo), which is the specific regulator for erythroid progenitor [erythrocytic burst-forming unit (BFU-E) and CFU-E] proliferation and differentiation (5). Growth factors for granulocyte-monocyte progenitors (CFU-GM) (6), megakaryocyte progenitors (CFU-Meg) (7), and lymphocyte progenitors (CFU-L) have also been reported (8,9).

A wide variety of cell types have been proposed to be involved in the cellular regulation of hemopoiesis. Monocytes and macrophages are thought to be important regulatory cells for lymphohemopoiesis. Those cells are also important accessory cells for a variety of immunological reactions (10). Macrophages are also involved in the regulation of myelopoiesis. A "nurse cell" function of macrophages for erythropoiesis has been inferred from the occurrence of "erythroblastic islands" (11). Monocytes and macrophages also produce a colony-stimulating factor (CSF) for *in vitro* granulocyte/macrophage colony formation (6). Studies by Kurland et al. (12–14) have demonstrated that monocytes and macrophages also produce prostaglandin E, which is an inhibitor of CFU-GM (13).

Lymphocytes, and specifically T lymphocytes, are also thought to be major cellular regulators for lymphohemopoiesis. Lymphocytes, for example, release lymphokines, including several classes of CSFs (15). Lymphokines are glycosylated polypeptide hormones produced by lymphocytes undergoing proliferative response to antigen or lectin. Lymphokine-associated CSFs for CFU-GM (16), CFU-Mix (17), CFU-E (4) have been described. In addition, activated T lymphocytes produce fibroblast growth factor, which may be important in pathological states such as myelofibrosis (18).

Other more controversial factors hypothesized to be involved in the regulation of stem and progenitor cell growth and differentiation are various stromal elements that are thought to exert microenvironmental influences (19–24). Such stromal factors were originally termed the hemopoietic inductive microenvironment by Trenton (19). It was proposed that they "induced" the differentiation of pluripotent hemopoietic stem cells (CFU-S) into specific commitment pathways of lymphohemopoiesis. However, recent evidence suggesting influence of humoral regulators or primitive stem cells has raised doubt as to the regulatory role of stromal elements on stem and progenitor cell differentiation. Nonetheless, evidence obtained from *in vivo* studies suggests a role for stromal cell influence in the regulation of hemopoiesis. (Such evidence is reviewed in detail in another section of this chapter.)

It is apparent from the model (Fig. 1) that the characterization of mechanisms involved in physiological and pathological (toxicity) states of hemopoiesis would be facilitated by techniques that provide concurrent evaluation of the quantitative and functional status of stem and progenitor cells, of the humoral and cellular regulators of those populations (including stromal components), and of the functional mature effector cells. Myelotoxic agents that affect essentially all levels of hemopoietic development have been described.

METHODS FOR THE STUDY OF MYELOTOXIC EFFECTS ON LYMPHOHEMOPOIETIC STEM AND PROGENITOR CELLS

The various assays for lymphohemopoietic stem and progenitor cells, humoral regulators, and candidate stromal microenvironmental components are outlined in Table 1. Methods for the *in vivo* study of pluripotent hemopoietic stem cells are first discussed in deference to historic considerations. Although the exact morphology of pluripotent stem cells is not known, results of studies on highly enriched gradient fractions of stem cells suggest a morphological "candidate" for pluripotent stem cells (25). Exclusive of morphological features, pluripotent stem cells can be studied and quantitated with assays that incorporate the basic criteria for their dual functions of self-maintenance and pluripotentiality. The standard assay for pluripotent stem cells is the spleen colony technique of Till and McCulloch (3). The investigators demonstrated that the intravenous injection of cells obtained from hemopoietic organs into lethally irradiated syngeneic mice resulted in the formation of discrete hemopoietic colonies in the spleen after about 7 days.

TABLE 1. *Summary of assays for measurement of hemopoietic stem and progenitor cells*

Potentiality of stem cells	Type of stem cell	Method	Stimulant
Pluripotent hemopoietic stem cells	CFU-S	*In vivo* spleen colony formation by reconstitution of lethally irradiated mice (3)	Mouse environment
		In vitro growth of CFU-S in suspension cultures (23,169–174)	Adherent stromal cells
Pluripotent stem cells with limited self-renewal	CFU-Mix	Formation of mixed hemopoietic colonies in agar or plasma clots (17,160–162)	Growth factors from mitogen-stimulated lymphocytes
Primitive erythrocytic committed stem cells	BFU-E	Plasma clot or agar and methylcellulose (77–79,85)	Epo (?), erythroid burst-promoting factor
		Long-term suspension cultures (23,169–174)	Adherent stromal cells
Committed erythrocytic progenitor cells	CFU-E	Plasma clot or methylcellulose semisolid culture systems (4,5,85,86)	Epo
		Long-term suspension cultures (23,169–174)	Adherent stromal cells
Granulocytic primitive committed stem cells	CFU-D	Diffusion chamber or diffusion chamber with agar (36,37, 71–75)	Mouse environment
Committed monocyte-granulocytic and/or macrophage progenitor cells	CFU-GM	Semisolid agar or methylcellulose culture systems (6,32,33,38–64)	CSF-GM conditioned media with human cell lines, human hairy cell leukemia, embryo cells, blood cells, PHA-stimulated lymphocytes, urine, serum
		Long-term suspension cultures (23,169–174)	Adherent stromal cells
Committed megakaryocytic progenitor cells	CFU-Meg	Semisolid agar cultures, plasma clot (7,34,88–95)	PHA-LyCM erythropoietin preparation
Committed lymphocytic progenitor cells	CFU-BL	Semisolid agar (9,129–141) culture systems	PHA-LyCM, PWM, 2-ME, protein A
	CFU-TL	Semisolid agar or methylcellulose cultures (8,101–128)	PHA and PWM alloantigens, T-dependent soluble antigens and TCGF
		T-Cell suspension long-term suspension cultures (10,15, 142,109,110)	TCGF
"Multipoiential" stromal "stem" cells and hemopoietic microenvironment		Inoculation of fibroblasts isolated from hemopoietic tissues into I.P. implanted diffusion chambers or directly into the renal capsule (22, 180,191)	*In vivo* mouse environment
Fibroblast progenitor cells	CFU-F	Formation of adherent fibroblast colonies in suspension or semisolid culture systems (22,24,178, 187–193)	Fibroblast growth factors(?), 2 ME, leukemic serum

Abbreviations: CFU-S, spleen colony-forming unit; CFU-GM, granulocyte/monocyte CFU; BFU-E, erythrocytic burst-forming unit; CFU-E, erythrocytic CFU; CFU-Meg, megakaryocytic CFU; CSF-GM, colony-stimulating factor for granulocyte/monocytes; PHA-LyCm, phytohemagglutinin-stimulated lymphocyte-conditioned medium; CFU-BL, B-lymphocyte CFU; CFU-TL, T-lymphocyte CFU; PB, precursor of B-lymphoid cells; TCGF, T-cell growth factor; PWM, pokeweed mitogen; Epo, erythropoietin.

The relationship of the number of cells injected and the number of resultant spleen colonies specifies the quantity of pluripotent stem cells (CFU-S). In the assay, erythroblastic, granulocytic, megakaryocytic, and mixed colonies are formed. Morphological lymphocytic colonies are not apparent, but transplantation of cells derived from the various myeloid colonies into lethally irradiated recipients results in reconstitution of immunocytes as well as myeloid elements (26).

Till and McCulloch demonstrated that spleen colonies developed by clonogenic proliferation from single stem cells (3). Further, self-replicative capacity and pluripotentiality of the spleen colony progenitors were also demonstrated, thus fulfilling the criterion for pluripotent hematopoietic stem cells (27). Thus, with reservations previously noted by Cronkite (*this volume*), the CFU-S assay has become the accepted method for the quantitation of pluripotent hemopoietic stem cells.

No techniques equivalent to the spleen colony assay for studies on pluripotent stem cells exist for species other than mice and rats. Focal proliferations resembling spleen colonies have been observed in the bone marrow of dogs recovering from radiation and reconstituted with bone marrow (28). However, as is discussed elsewhere in this chapter, recent techniques have been developed that allow for the continuous growth of pluripotent hemopoietic stem cells in liquid cultures from humans (29) and other species (30,31), and clonal culture methods have been described that allow for the growth of "stem cells" with at least limited capacity for self-renewal and with pluripotent differentiation capacities (17) (Table 1).

Although the spleen colony assay has provided an important method for investigating the pluripotent hemopoietic stem cell, a major disadvantage is that the technique is principally limited to studies on rodents. Thus, the introduction of clonal methods allowing for the growth of the variety of lymphohemopoietic progenitor cells in semisolid culture systems provided a major new approach for the investigation of myelotoxicity in a wide variety of animal species, including humans.

In 1966 Bradley and Metcalf (32) and Pluznik and Sachs (33) reported that when hemopoietic cells are immobilized in semisolid media (agar) in the presence of appropriate growth factors, subsequent incubation resulted in the formation of colonies composed of differentiated hemopoietic cells. Such colonies were composed of cells of the granulocytic and monocyte-macrophage series. Colony formation was shown to be dependent on granulocyte-macrophage colony-stimulating factor (GM-CSF) and was clonogenic in origin, resulting from repeated cell divisions and cellular differentiation. The undifferentiated precursor of such colonies (clones) was termed a colony-forming unit in culture (CFU-C) or, more recently, CFU-GM. Studies demonstrated that such progenitor cells were not pluripotent stem cells (i.e., CFU-S equivalents) but rather their descendants, which were committed to specific lines of cellular differentiation. Thus, they were termed committed stem cells or, more appropriately, progenitor cells. Subsequently, methods for the *in vitro* growth of committed progenitors for essentially all lines of lymphohemopoietic progenitor have been described (Table 1) (1). In those assays single cells that are immobilized in semisolid media such as agar, plasma clot, or methylcellulose are induced to proliferate by various specific growth factors or mitogens. Repeated division of such target cells results ultimately in the production of various specifically differentiated lymphohemopoietic colonies that can be quantitated. Techniques exist for the growth of committed progenitors for CFU-GM (6), candidate "stromal" progenitors for fibroblast (CFU-F) (22), erythroid progenitors (CFU-E, BFU-E) (4,5), megakaryocyte progenitors (CFU-Meg) (34), eosinophil progenitors (35), T-lymphocyte progenitors (CFU-T) (8), B-lymphocyte progenitors (CFU-BL) (9), primitive granulocyte-monocyte progenitors in diffusion chambers (CFU-D) (36,37), mixed hemopoietic colonies (17) (CFU-mix, possible pluripotent stem cells with limited self-replicative capacity), and "presumptive" human hemopoietic stem cells (Ia-resistant-CFU-C) (29). The morphological appearance of macrophage and T-lymphocyte colonies is shown in Figs. 2 and 3, respectively.

Although colonies in the various classes consist of mature lymphohemopoietic effector cells, they are ultimately clonally derived from a single undifferentiated progenitor cell. Thus the clonal assays provide methods for the simultaneous investigation of myelotoxic effects produced both on cellular proliferation (amplification) and on cellular differentiation. In addition, since the various culture systems have an absolute requirement for specific growth factors (such as Epo for red blood cell colony formation), the clonal methods can also be used to evaluate toxic effects produced on various hemopoietic humoral regulators or populations responsible for their production.

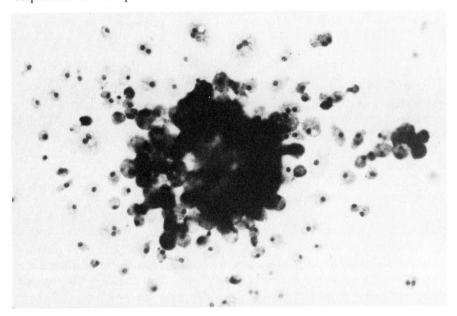

FIG. 2. Murine bone marrow macrophage colony ($\times$400).

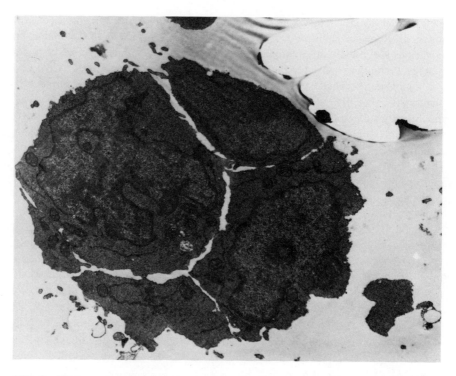

FIG. 3. Electron micrograph of a human mixed-lymphocyte stimulated T-lymphocyte colony grown in agarose (×16,000).

TECHNIQUES FOR GRANULOCYTE/MACROPHAGE COLONIES

Methods for the *in vitro* clonogenic growth of committed granulocyte/macrophage progenitors are reviewed first, as these populations were historically the first to be described. Bradley and Metcalf (32) and Pluznik and Sachs (33) reported that incubation of hemopoietic cells, immobilized in semisolid media such as agar gels and in the presence of appropriate growth factors, resulted in the formation of colonies composed of differentiated hemopoietic cells. Such colonies were composed of differentiated cells of the granulocytic and monocyte-macrophage series. Such colonies were demonstrated as clonogenic in origin and derived from a unipotential, undifferentiated progenitor cell committed to granulocyte/macrophage differentiation pathways. The progenitor is termed CFU for granulocyte-macrophages or CFU-GM (1). Colony formation by CFU-GM involves both proliferation and differentiation of the progenitors with consequent development of functionally mature granulocytes and macrophages. Both processes (proliferation/differentiation) were demonstrated as absolutely dependent on a source of growth factor(s) termed granulocyte-monocyte CSF or GM-CSF (6). Such molecular species were subsequently shown to consist of a family of glycoproteins with variable propensity for inducing proliferation and/or differentiation of CFU-GM (6,38–47).

Over the past decade numerous studies on the characterization of CFU-GM and GM-CSF have been reported (6,46–55). Despite intensive experimental investigation, the role of GM-CSF as a true *in vivo* physiological regulator of granulopoiesis (i.e., granulopoietin) *in vivo* has not been unequivocally established.

Although the clonogenic growth of granulocyte/macrophage colonies was originally described for murine species (32,33), methods for the assay of CFU-GM are currently available for a wide variety of experimental animals and for humans (48).

Numerous studies have demonstrated that CFU-GM are not pluripotent hemopoietic stem cells (CFU-S), as they are neither pluripotent nor self-replicative but rather represent biopotential descendants of CFU-S, which are specifically "committed" to specific lines of cellular differentiation for granulocytes and monocyte/macrophages (1,32,33,38–47,49,50).

In addition to their limited differentiation capacity for granulocyte/macrophage development, evidence that CFU-GM are populations distinct from CFU-S comes from a variety of experiments, including their response to ^{3}H-Tdr suicide (49), density gradient profiles (50), and comparisons of the response of CFU-S and CFU-GM in animals subjected to bone marrow insults or manifesting various hemopoietic disorders (51–53).

Thus, dividing stem cells have the "choice" of forming progeny that retain stem cell properties (self-replication and pluripotentiality) or progeny that differentiate into progenitor cells with sequentially limited capacities for self-replication, proliferation, and pluripotentiality and ultimately to form nondividing end cells.

It is generally known that GM-CSF is a glycoprotein that induces extensive proliferation and differentiation of myeloid progenitor cells *in vitro* (6). Incubation of this factor with bone marrow cells in semisolid gels leads to the development of granulocyte and macrophage colonies. The initial step involved in the action of GM-CSF on responsive cells seems to bind this factor to membrane receptors as observed by incubation and autoradiographic studies (45–47).

Several lines of evidence indicate that GM-CSF is required continuously for colony development (55). Exposure of marrow cells to GM-CSF for short intervals does not lead to subsequent colony formation (55), whereas the transfer of early cells or clusters that have been exposed to GM-CSF for 2 to 4 days into new median devoid of GM-CSF results in a decline in cell number and colony formation (56). In addition, GM-CSF is known to induce RNA and protein synthesis in mature granulocytes (57) and to induce mature macrophages to become tumoricidal (58). This suggests that GM-CSF may act on mature cells as well as on progenitor cells by initiating intracellular program for both proliferative and differentiative cell functions.

Current evidence suggests the presence of at least three major classes of specific CSF effecting proliferation and differentiation of CFU-GM. The three subclasses of murine GM-CSF have been purified to homogeneity by Metcalf (54). Interactions between the three regulators influence the degree of proliferative and granulocyte and/or monocyte-macrophage differentiation from principally bipotential CFU-GM.

Commitment to either differentiation pathway is irreversible, requires one to two complete cell cycles in the presence of the regulator, and is an asymmetrical event.

Studies by Stanley and others (59–63) also indicate that several growth factors are involved in the production of mononuclear phagocytes from CFU-S. The major regulator is colony-stimulating factor (CSF-1), which specifically regulates the survival, proliferation, and differentiation of cells of the mononuclear phagocytic lineage (59–60). CSF-1 can be detected by specific radioimmunoassays and radioreceptor assays (61). It is a glycoprotein consisting of two similar disulfide-bonded subunits with N-glycosidically linked acidic "complex" carbohydrate moieties (62). Specific cell surface receptors for CSF-1 occur only on mononuclear phagocytic cells. They mediate the biological effects as well as the degradation of the growth factor (63). These receptors are excellent markers of mononuclear phagocytes irrespective of their state of differentiation or tissue of origin.

CFU-GM inhibitory factors have also been described (64). It has been proposed that the stimulatory effects of GM-CSF on CFU-GM are counteracted by at least two negative regulators: prostaglandin E (PGE) and acidic isoferritin. For example, monocytes and macrophages produce PGE, which is inhibitory to CFU-GM (12,13). Since monocytes and macrophages are also sources for the production of GM-CSF, Kurland (14) proposed a unique regulatory role of monocytes and macrophages in the positive-negative regulation of granulopoiesis.

Numerous studies have demonstrated the direct effects of myelotoxic agents on CFU-GM (53,65–67). In addition, recent studies have indicated that some myelotoxic chemicals can also affect or interfere with the action of GM-CSF on progenitor cells (68–70).

For example, chloramphenicol (a drug with known myelotoxic potential in humans) has been reported to inhibit the growth of CFU-GM (68). The inhibition of colony formation was prevented by increasing the concentration of GM-CSF to the culture medium. Although chloramphenicol also inhibited the growth of erythroid colonies (CFU-E), the inhibitory effect of the drug was not reversed by increasing concentrations of Epo (69).

More recently, Pigoli et al. (70) observed similar "sparing" effects of GM-CSF on CFU-GM toxicity produced by vindesine (VDS). VDS is a semisynthetic vinca-alkaloid related to vinblastine and vincristine, which have similar mechanisms of actions: They inhibit microtubule formation during the mitotic phase of the cell cycle. A dose-dependent inhibition of granulocyte-macrophage colony formation was observed with increasing doses of VDS using murine bone marrow. Further, addition of anti-CSF serum during preincubation abolished the protective effect of GM-CSF (70). Whereas inhibition of CFU-GM was produced when using 100 units of GM-CSF, no inhibition of colony formation occurred at the same dose of VDS when 200 units of GM-CSF were used. Preincubation of cells with VDS and CSF also prevented inhibition that occurred with VDS alone.

A second method for the growth of granulocyte monocyte-macrophage progenitors is the diffusion chamber technique primarily described by Boyum and Borgstrom (36).

The diffusion-chamber technique deserves special consideration with respect to the study of myelotoxicity in humans. For obvious reasons, such studies are largely limited to *in vitro* approaches or extrapolations must be made from data on *in vivo* exposures in experimental animals (with the limited exception of myelotoxic agents used clinically such as chemotheraputic agents). *In vitro* exposure of human cells has a major limitation as it does not reflect the continuous changes that occur *in vivo* as a result of biometabolism and biodegradation. *In vitro* studies are not usually possible for chemicals requiring biological activation such as cyclophosphamide (biological). In addition, no method for the *in vivo* assay of pluripotent hemopoietic stem cells exists for humans that is equivalent to the spleen colony assay (CFU-S) in rodents.

One approach to resolving the problems associated with *in vitro* chemical exposures and intraspecies extrapolations for studies on human myelotoxicity is the use of the agar diffusion-chamber assay previously described by Dr. Marsh (*this volume*) (36,37). The assay has the advantage of allowing for the exposure of human progenitor cells in an *in vivo* milieu and thus allows for studies on human cells of drugs requiring biometabolism and also reflects biodegradative changes. Thus, the method interfaces techniques for the clonal growth of hemopoietic progenitors in semisolid culture with an approach to allow studies of myelotoxicity of human cells in an *in vivo* environment. In addition, studies have indicated that the progenitor cells for the formation CFU-D are more primitive than the CFU-GM, representing a progenitor at least as primitive as a cell intermediate to CFU-S and CFU-GM (37).

The technique originally described by Boyum and Borgstrom (36) involved the use of single cells but was later adapted to a semisolid agar culture system by Gordon et al. (71). Briefly, bone marrow cells suspended in agar medium are introduced into cell-impermeable diffusion chambers that are subsequently incubated in the peritoneal cavity of recipient host mice. For human bone marrow studies, host mice are previously irradiated (900 rad, $^{60}Co,\gamma$-radiation) to provide an environment conclusive to colony formation. Nonirradiated mice provide adequate environments for the formation of CFU-D for mouse bone marrow. Following removal of the diffusion chambers, the formation of granulocyte colonies are scored following 8 to 9 days incubation in the peritoneal environment.

Since human CFU-D can be grown in the peritoneal cavity of mice, the technique therefore allows for the study of drugs or chemicals requiring bioactivation and for the observation of chemical changes due to biodegradation. In addition, the comparison of *in vitro* dose-response relationships of CFU-D for human and marine targets provides data on species variables and allows for the extrapolation of results obtained for murine *in vivo* studies to humans.

An example of the usefulness and application of the diffusion-chamber technique to the investigation of human myelotoxicity is provided by the studies of Marsh (*this volume*) and Gordon et al. (72–74). Gorden et al. studied the effect of a single high dose of cyclophosphamide on human bone marrow CFU-D and compared dose-response relationships obtained for human and mouse CFU-D exposed *in vitro* to the drug. They simultaneously determined the effect of the drug for mouse CFU-D exposed *in situ* in the bone marrow. In addition, changes in the proliferation rate of CFU-D were studied by monitoring their response to the S-phase specific drug cytosine arabinoside (Ara-C).

The authors compared the sensitivity of human and mouse bone marrow CFU-D supported by diffusion chambers placed into mice subjected to graded doses of cyclophosphamide (72–74). Under these conditions human CFU-D were found to be far more sensitive to cyclophosphamide than were CFU-D in mouse marrow implants. However, mouse CFU-D were found to be equally sensitive whether exposures were done on cells contained in diffusion chambers or on CFU-D *in situ* in the bone marrow. The later observations suggest that for cyclophosphamide the assay of CFU-D in the peritoneal cavity is a good indication of toxicity of CFU-D *in situ*.

These studies (72–74) and those previously described (Marsh, *this volume*) demonstrate that the diffusion chamber technique can be used as a model for the study of human primitive progenitor cells for drugs requiring *in vivo* biological activation and allows compensation for changes in the drug occurring from biodegradation.

The other important issue related to the CFU-D assay is that it provides an assay for human progenitor cells that are more primitive than the classic committed progenitor cells for granulocyte-macrophage differentiation pathways (CFU-GM). Even though CFU-D give rise to only granulocytic elements in the diffusion chamber, they have pluripotent differentiation capacities on retransplantation (37).

Numerous studies have indicated differences between CFU-D and CFU-GM and, conversely, a close relationship of CFU-D to CFU-S (37,75). For example, recent studies by Niskamen (75) examined the parent-progeny relationship between murine CFU-S and CFU-D. In these studies individual colonies forming in diffusion chambers containing mouse bone marrow were removed following 5 and 8 days of incubation in the mouse peritoneal cavity. Cells retrieved from individual colonies were subsequently injected into lethally irradiated mice and the formation of spleen colonies (CFU-S, 8 or 12 days postinjection) was determined.

Seventy-five percent of day 5 CFU-D colonies gave rise to day 12 spleen colonies and 13% to day 8 CFU-S. Day 8 CFU-D gave rise to 63% and 23% CFU-S on day 12 and 8, respectively. In reverse experiments the formation of diffusion chamber colonies from cells obtained from individual spleen colonies was investigated. Day 8 and day 12 spleen colonies gave rise in order to 0% and 30% day 5 CFU-D. None of the CFU-S colonies gave rise to day 8 CFU-D. The authors concluded (75) that the majority of the cells that gave rise to colonies in diffusion chambers (CFU-D) on day 5 were at least as primitive as day 12 CFU-S and that since some day 12 CFU-S gave rise to day 5 CFU-D, the precursors of the two colony types (*in vivo* and *in vitro*) may be identical.

ERYTHROID COLONIES

Until the development of *in vitro* clonogenic techniques for the growth of erythroid progenitors, regulatory mechanisms of erythropoiesis were studied mainly *in vivo*. The primary humoral regulator of erythropoiesis is Epo, as demonstrated by its ability to stimulate proliferation of erythroid progenitor cells and its ability to induce erythroid maturation as reflected by hemoglobin synthesis. Prior to the advent of *in vitro* erythroid cloning techniques, the effects of Epo were studied using *in vivo* methods such as the stimulation of hemoglobin synthesis as measured by ^{59}Fe incorporation (76). The target cells for Epo in such systems were defined as the erythropoietin-responsive cell (ERC). The ERCs were considered to be primitive hemopoietic cells, not morphologically recognizable as erythroid but that which undergoes proliferation and differentiation with hemoglobin synthesis in response to Epo.

The development of methods allowing for the *in vitro* clonogenic growth of various classes of Epo-responsive progenitors has greatly facilitated studies on mechanisms involved in the regulation of erythropoiesis (4,5,77–86). Since both *in vivo* and *in vitro* techniques are available to study erythroid progenitors, studies on erythropoiesis are enhanced relative to the investigation of granulopoiesis, which is mainly limited to *in vitro* approaches. In addition, although the physiological role of Epo in the humoral regulation of erythropoiesis is firmly established, the proposed regulator(s) of granulopoiesis (CFU-GM) is still largely hypothetical.

Currently, semisolid culture systems are available for the clonogenic growth of at least two major classes of erythroid progenitors in semisolid culture systems in the presence of Epo (4,5,77–86). Such techniques are available for humans (84), as well as for experimental animals (4,5). By manipulating culture conditions, several subpopulations of erythroid progenitors can be identified based on differential sensitivity to Epo, proliferation potential, culture interval, cell-cycle characteristics, physical characteristics, and responsiveness to *in vivo* manipulation of erythropoiesis (85).

Variation of Epo concentration and time in culture identifies two major classes of erythroid progenitors. Stephenson et al. (5) reported that colonies of hemoglobin synthesizing cells in cultures of mouse bone marrow cells stimulated by Epo formed following 2 days of incubation. The progenitor of the 2-day erythroid colonies was termed CFU-E for erythroid colony-forming unit (5).

By the 10th day of incubation in the presence of high concentrations of Epo, large erythroid colonies containing reticulocytes and erythrocytes form, the progenitor of which were termed burst-forming units (BFU-E) by Axelrad et al. (77,78) owing to their explosive growth characteristics and large colonies. The BFU-E can form colonies containing up to 10^4 cells (79) that eventually differentiate into reticulocytes, which impart a bright red gross appearance to the bursts (85). In addition, large cells resembling megakaryocytes can be observed within the erythroid bursts (4). The incidence of the erythroid progenitors in mouse bone marrow is approximately $150/10^5$ nucleated cells for CFU-E and $30/10^5$ nucleated cells for BFU-E (85). One major difference between BFU-E and CFU-E is the relatively high levels of Epo required for burst formation. Contrary to erythroid colony formation, burst formation is characterized by a delay of approximately 6 days, which may suggest that BFU-E does not respond directly to Epo (4,85).

In addition to BFU-E and CFU-E, intermediate forms of erythroid progenitors can be observed by variation in incubation time. For example, Wagemaker et al. (85) reported the formation of small numbers of erythroid clusters following 3 to 4 days incubation (termed 3- or 4-day BFU-E). Such progenitors were thought to be intermediate in differentiation characteristics to BFU-E and CFU-E (85).

Considerable evidence has indicated that BFU-E are more primitive erythroid progenitors than are CFU-E. This is based on proliferative status, cell-cycle and physical characteristics, relationship to CFU-S response to Epo, and *in vivo* responsiveness to experimental manipulations of erythropoiesis (5,77–85).

Hemoglobin synthesis does not begin in the largest and most primitive of the colonies (BFU-E) until 8 to 10 days, implying that extensive proliferation of BFU-E without differentiation is occurring. The various erythroid progenitors also differ in physical properties such as their sedimentation velocities (85). BFU-E have a sedimentation rate that coincides with that of pluripotent stem cells (CFU-S) while day 3 BFU-E apparently are intermediate between BFU-E and CFU-E (85). The sensitivity to Epo also suggests a similar sequential differentiation sequence for the three progenitors (82,85).

Although Epo as well as serum are the major limiting factors for the growth of both BFU-E and CFU-E, studies have suggested that BFU-E (unlike CFU-E) are not directly responsive to Epo (4,82,85). For example, BFU-E can survive and probably proliferate in the absence of Epo (4) whereas the Epo requirement for CFU-E is similar for both *in vitro* and *in vivo* environments (77,82). This relationship does not hold for BFU-E. Whereas the serum requirement of CFU-E can be explained (probably entirely) on the basis of their defined requirements for albumin, transferrin, and lipid, the serum requirements of BFU-E cannot (4). High concentrations of Epo are required for BFU-E colony formation *in vitro* (4,77,82), but such Epo dependency is not seen for BFU-E in the intact mouse. Thus, BFU-E colony formation is not responsive to *in vivo* manipulations of Epo (i.e., sustained elevation or suppression of Epo by anemia, hypoxia, or hypertransfusion) (82), but are clearly under influence of Epo-independent mechanisms (4,82). On the basis of these and other observations, it has been suggested that Epo is required only for the latter stages of development of BFU-E, serving primarily to render colonies recognizable as erythroid by initiating hemoglobin synthesis. In addition, in view of the unique serum dependency of BFU-E, it has been proposed that a specific serum factor is essential for the proliferation and differentiation of BFU-E (4,81–85).

Several studies have indicated the existence of serum or cellular-derived factor(s) that enhances the growth of BFU-E (4,85). Wagemaker et al. (85,86) showed a dependency on a bone-marrow-associated factor for the growth and differentiation of BFU-E in the presence of Epo. Similar burst-promoting activity (BPA) was observed in fetal calf and horse serum (85), and BPA was observed in the serum of mice subjected to severe hemopoietic stress (85) and in media conditioned by human peripheral blood leukocytes (85).

It is of interest that human-leukocyte-conditioned media not only exhibit BPA-like activity on murine BFU-E, but additionally initiate DNA synthesis in pluripotent stem cells (CFU-S) and induce CSF responsiveness in a distinct, low-density subpopulation of CFU-C (85,87).

In more recent studies, Iscove (4) described the stimulation of Epo-independent growth of early erythroid progenitors by BPA produced by media conditioned by lectin-stimulated mouse spleen cells. The studies presented evidence that (a) Epo is required for the late but not early stages of colony formation by BFU-E, (b) molecules in conditioned media (glycoproteins with an apparent molecular weight of 3,500) by lectin-stimulated spleen cells can replace much of the serum requirements for early but not late stages of colony formation by BFU-E, (c) BPA reduced the threshold requirements of Epo for burst formation and that BPA also induced the formation of mixed colonies composed of both erythroid and granulocytic cells. BPA was further observed to increase the number of large cells, presumably megakaryocytes in erythroid colonies (4). The authors suggested that BPA may represent a new class of humoral regulator(s) operating not only on committed erythroid progenitors but also at the level of pluripotent stem cells (4,85).

Thus, it appears that similar to the dependency for the functional survival of CFU-E (but not BFU-E) on Epo, BPA is essential for the survival of BFU-E but not CFU-E. BPA also appears to promote colony formation by cells having pluripotent differentiation capacity for erythrocytes, granulocytes, and megakaryocytes (see subsequent section on mixed colonies on CFU-Mix). BPA actions appear to be restricted to early hemopoietic precursors—pluripotent and at least primitive-committed erythroid progenitors (4,85).

MEGAKARYOCYTE COLONIES

Blood platelet production is essential for the initiation of hemostasis and the maintenance of the integrity of the blood vasculature. Platelets are derived from megakaryocytes, which are largely nonproliferative. Thus, populations of megakaryocytic progenitors capable of cellular amplification are essential to the maintenance of thrombocyte hemostasis. Methods are currently available for the assay of committed megakaryocyte progenitors (CFU-Meg) by the growth of megakaryocyte colonies in plasma cultures (7,88) or semisolid agar (N3,4,5) (89–91) in the presence of specific growth factor(s) (thrombopoietin). Studies on megakaryocyte progenitors are complicated by the fact that megakaryocyte precursors are capable of both cellular division as well as endoreduplication (nuclear replication without cell division or endomitosis), and as a consequence the existence of both diploid (2N) and polypoid (4N to 32N) progenitors is theoretically possible (92).

Nonetheless, the development of various methods for the detection and investigation of megakaryocyte progenitors *in vitro* has provided a major new approach for the study of megakaryocytopoiesis and for the detection of agents producing adverse effects on platelet production. Techniques for the growth of megakaryocyte colonies in semisolid cultures using blood plasma (7,88) and agar (90,91) were originally described for the mouse. Methods for the assay of human CFU-Meg were later reported (92).

Nakeff et al. (7) first reported the clonogenic growth of megakaryocyte colonies from mouse bone marrow using a plasma culture system. Briefly, the method involved the growth of bone marrow cells in bovine citrated plasma, tissue culture medium, horse serum, and spleen-conditioned medium. The last serves as a source of CSF and is produced by stimulation of spleen cells with pokeweed mitogen. Following 4 days incubation and staining for the cytoplasmic marker acetylcholinesterase (AChE), colonies containing four or more AChE-positive cells are counted as reflecting the number of CFU-Meg present.

The AChE-positive cells in the colonies are composed of megakaryocytes in various stages of maturation, and studies by McLeod et al. (89) demonstrated electron microscopic evidence of platelet formation in plasma clot cultures containing Epo. Other studies have indicated that CFU-Meg are positive for platelet antigen (93), are nonphagocytic (92), and nonadherent (92).

Numerous studies have been done on the proliferative capacity, physiochemical characterization, and differentiation potentials of CFU-Meg (7,88–95). Studies have been done on cell size of the progenitors using unit velocity sedimentation (90) and on cell density using discontinuous albumin gradient centrifugation (94).

As studies have indicated that the morphologically recognizable megakaryocytes are largely nonproliferating cells, the progenitor cell compartments undoubtedly are major components, for the cellular amplification component of platelet production occurs in response to physiological demand. Nakeff (95) and Nakeff and Bryan (92) conducted studies attempting to characterize the capacity of CFU-Meg for cellular proliferation and endomitosis as reflected in the ploidy level. Based on the response to "survive" high doses of S-phase specific agents (hydroxyurea and Ara-C) it was estimated that in mouse bone marrow 15% to 20% and 40% to 50% of CFU-Meg are not active in DNA synthesis *in vivo* and *in vitro*, respectively.

A critical issue regarding the *in vitro* growth of megakaryocyte colonies is to what extent do they respond to proposed normal physiological regulations of megakaryocytopoiesis and platelet production. Studies have suggested that platelet production and megakaryocyte progenitor proliferation are under humoral regulation and that serum from platelet-depleted mice contains a factor(s) (thrombopoietin) that may stimulate the production of new megakaryocytes (96). It is also known that proliferation and differentiation of CFU-Meg are dependent on the presence of megakaryocyte colony-stimulating activity (Meg-CSA).

The serum of acutely immune-induced thrombocytopenic mice has been demonstrated to contain a high titer of thrombopoietin approximately 12 hours following acute platelet depletion as determined by an *in vivo* radiobioassay (95).

Nakeff and Bryan (92) therefore studied the effect of thrombopoietin, obtained from the serum of mice with immune-induced thrombocytopenia, on the incidence of CFU-Meg in bone marrow 12 hours after the injection of rabbit antimouse platelet gamma globulin (RAMP-g6). The addition of up to 20% thrombopoietin to bone marrow cultures resulted in an approximate doubling in the incidence of CFU-Meg.

Also, the effect with time of immune-induced thrombocytopenia in bone marrow CFU-M was compared with effects on blood platelets and marrow megakaryocytes (92). It was found that in response to severe demands for platelet production, a rapid sequence of compensatory changes was seen in all parameters, starting first with an increase in the CFU-Meg compartment, followed by changes in the small AChE-positive progenitors, and finally affecting mature megakaryocytes with ultimate restoration of normal peripheral blood platelet values. The studies indicate both *in vitro* and *in vivo* effects of thrombopoietin on CFU-Meg proliferation and further imply that CFU-Meg respond to demands for peripheral blood platelet production. These effects appear to be mediated by a humoral regulator (thrombopoietin) that appears, in part, to stimulate CFU-Meg proliferation and possibly differentiation.

Other attempts at ascribing a role of CFU-Meg in the physiological regulation of megakaryocytopoiesis include studies on the characterization of CFU-Meg in mice of W/W^v and Sl/Sl^d genotypes (92,97–99). Mice of strains W/W^v and Sl/Sl^d represent two classes of genetically anemic mice owing to defects occurring in pluripotent hemopoietic stem cells or to microenvironmental factors, respectively (97). In addition to anemia, both strains of mice have demonstrated abnormalities in megakaryocytes despite normal peripheral blood platelet numbers (98,99). It was found that both W/W^v and Sl/Sl^d mice have reduced numbers of CFU-Meg in the bone marrow relative to their normal congenic litter mates.

Studies in humans have also produced evidence for the existence of a humoral regulator of megakaryocytopoiesis. Mazur et al. (100) demonstrated that the sera of aplastic anemia patients contain an activity (Meg-CSA) that promotes proliferation and differentiation of CFU-Meg *in vitro*. The aplastic anemia was produced in response to five courses of intensive antileukemic chemotherapy. Elevations in Meg-CSA were first observed 4 to 7 days after initiating chemotherapy and at a time when thrombocytopenia was developing. Elevations in Meg-CSA of up to fourfold over base-line levels were observed even though platelet counts were maintained above 100,000/mm^3. Meg-CSA usually was observed to return to baseline levels prior to normalization of thrombocytes. Platelet transfusions resulted in depression of Meg-CSA. The authors concluded that Meg-CSA is a potent humoral megakaryocyte progenitor cell regulator that can be induced by intensive chemotherapy (100).

An example of the use of the CFU-Meg assay for the detection of selective toxicity to megakaryocyte progenitors is provided by the studies of Nakeff (92) on the effects of hydroxyurea and in Ara-C and CFU-S, CFU-E. The studies were actually done to determine the proliferative status of that fraction of CFU-Meg in DNA synthesis by using S-phase specific drugs (i.e., high-dose suicide). Their results on survival data demonstrated that the fraction of CFU-Meg in DNA synthesis is closer to CFU-S than to CFU-E. The latter are known to be more differentiated and mostly in cell cycle (92).

LYMPHOCYTE COLONIES

The development of techniques for the production of monoclonal antibodies has received much attention as a major new method for the characterization of humoral immunity and for the production of highly specific monoclonal antibodies. Methods for the *in vitro* growth of T-lymphocyte clones have received far less attention. The ability to grow functional clones of T lymphocytes (monoclonal T lymphocytes) could prove to be as valuable to studies on cellular immunology as monoclonal antibodies have been to investigations of humoral immunity.

Methods for the quantitation of lymphocyte blastogenesis based on the measurement of uptake of radiolabeled DNA precursors such as [3]HTdr have been utilized for many years in studies on cellular immunology. Consequently, the techniques have been extensively refined to allow for routine semi-automated quantitation of lymphocyte blastogenesis induced by T-cell (or B-cell) mitogens. It is therefore appropriate to ask if it is reasonable to pursue the development of methods for the growth of T-lymphocyte colonies that during their relative state of infancy appear to be less sophisticated, more laborious, and, indeed, redundant to standard methods for measuring lymphocyte stimulation.

Several studies have demonstrated that the colony-forming assays are more sensitive for detecting alterations in lymphocyte blastogenesis than are the DNA-precursor incorporation techniques (101-105, and F. D. Wilson, *unpublished data*). Increased sensitivity of the colony techniques has been reported for the quantitation of radiation effects (103), for the detection of serum suppressor activity in pregnant women (101), for the measurement of allogenic disparity (105), trace elemental toxicity (F. D. Wilson, *unpublished data*), and for the detection of T-cell clonal abnormalities in patients with Fanconi's anemia (102) and other hemopoietic disorders (104).

Several basic factors explain the increased sensitivity of colony techniques over the incorporation methods: [3]HTdr incorporation is an indirect measurement of cell division. DNA synthesis and consequent [3]HTdr incorporation can occur without subsequent cell division. In contrast, colony formation, by definition, requires actual and repeated cell division. Another major advantage of the colony method over the [3]HTdr-incorporation technique is that since individual colonies can be visualized, a potential means is provided for dissecting out and functionally characterizing clones of T lymphocytes.

Numerous techniques have been described for the growth of T- and B-lymphocyte colonies from both experimental animals and humans (8,9,101–159). A fundamental problem with T-lymphocyte colonies is whether or not they are truly clonal in origin. Studies indicating both a clonal origin (109,110) and a polyclonal genesis (143,144) have been reported. Facet and Testa (144), for example, conducted studies on the isoenzyme characteristics (glucose-6-phosphate dehydrogenase, G6PD) of T-lymphocyte colonies grown for a donor heterozygous for the enzyme. CFU-T-lymphocyte colonies contained both type A and B isoenzymes and thus were not monoclonal in origin. Based on the distribution pattern of isoenzyme electrophoretic bands, the authors concluded that an average of two T-lymphocyte clones proliferate per colony (144).

Singer et al. (145) also found T-lymphocyte colonies to be heterogeneous for G6PD isoenzymes. However, those authors further observed that when a promotor of T-cell colony growth (12-0-tetracecanoylphorbol 13-acetate, TPA) was added to cultures, the frequency of polyclonal colonies was reduced. The authors concluded that despite the apparent multicellular origin of T-cell colonies in cultures without TPA, monoclonal growth of T-cell colonies could be achieved by adding TPA when cultures were done at low colony densities. Reports demonstrating the establishment of antigen-specific clonal lines (109,110) suggest that at least under some culture conditions the development and isolation of monoclonal T-cell colonies in semisolid cultures are indeed possible. Moreover, regardless of their origin (monoclonal or polyclonal), numerous studies have indicated the T-lymphocyte colony techniques are far more sensitive for the detection of immunotoxic effects than are the standard methods for measuring lymphocyte blastogenesis by quantitation of incorporation of radiolabeled DNA precursors such as ^{3}HTdr (101–105).

Methods for the growth of murine and human T-lymphocyte colonies in semisolid culture systems were first described by Srendi et al. (8) and Rozenszain et al. (113), respectively. In the original methods, a two-step system in which the pre-sensitization of lymphocytes with T-cell mitogen was first required in liquid-phase culture prior to colony growth in semisolid culture (8,113). Subsequently, methods for the direct growth of T-lymphocyte colonies in one-step semisolid culture systems were described (111,114,124,125). Further, methods using single-layer (124) and double-layer (114) agar culture systems and the stimulation of T-cell colonies in response to mitogens [phytohemagglutinin (PHA), concanavalin A (ConA), and pokeweed mitogen (PWM)] and alloantigens (105,126,128) have been reported. The growth of peripheral blood T-lymphocyte colonies from gradient-enriched mononuclear cell factors (8,113,114,124,125) and directly from whole blood (103,112) is also possible.

The two-phase system originally described for the growth of human T-lympho-cyte colonies by Rozenszain et al. (113) was subsequently shown to result in cellular clumping, and, consequently, methods for the direct growth of T-lymphocyte colonies in agar without presensitization with mitogen in liquid-phase culture were developed (124). Although a wide variety of methods for the growth of T-cell colonies have been described, the basic requirements are similar for all systems. T-lymphocyte colony formation minimally requires the presence of a T-cell mitogen which can be a plant lectin such as PHA or ConA (106,111–125), alloantigens (105,126,139), or T-dependent soluable antigens such as purified protein derivative (PPD) (102,109,110).

Numerous studies have demonstrated a T-cell nature of the colonies (8,113,114,117,118,120,124,126). Colony cells form spontaneous rosettes with sheep erythrocytes (E-rosettes) and bear human T-lymphocyte antigen (146). In addition, T-lymphocyte colony cells have been demonstrated to have significant cytotoxic capacity of both antibody-dependent and antibody-independent types (147). T-cell colony formation has also been shown to develop from a T-cell subset rather than from null cells (148). Studies have suggested that PHA-induced colony cells possibly belong to the inducer/helper subset of T lymphocytes (149).

Studies have demonstrated enhanced T-lymphocyte colony formation by factors released from mitogen (PHA)-stimulated T lymphocytes [T-cell growth factor, (TCGF), interleukin II, lymphocyte colony-enhancing factor] (148). TCGF may be added to culture directly or in feeder layers in a double agar culture system (150).

In addition to growth factors released from mitogen-stimulated T cells, both stimulatory and inhibitory factors for T-lymphocyte colony growth have been shown to be released by macrophages (151). Srendi et al. (151), for example, investigated the effects of macrophages on mouse lymph node CFU-TL using culture supernatents obtained from spleen or peritoneal adherent macrophage populations. Both inhibitory and stimulatory factors for T-lymphocyte colony formation were observed. The lymphocyte colony-inhibitory factor concentrated in fractions with a molecular weight of less than 1,000 whereas the lymphocyte colony-enhancing factor was mainly located in the fraction having a molecular weight of 10,000 to 30,000. The inhibitory factor was heat stable whereas the colony-enhancing factor was not.

More recently, Klein et al. (121) conducted studies on the mechanism of action and on the nature of cooperating cells controlling human T-lymphocyte colony formation. Media conditioned by PHA-stimulated blood mononuclear cells were tested for their ability to stimulate T-cell colonies. Target cells were cellular populations remaining after treatment with anti(Fab')2 cell affinity chromotography of mononuclear cells. Population was demonstrated to contain CFU-TL but to be devoid of cells essential for promotion of T-cell colonies, thus requiring a feeder layer containing media conditioned by PHA-stimulated mononuclear cells in order to generate T-lymphocyte colonies. PHA was found to be necessary at least for two steps of T-colony formation: for the production of colony promotory activity by PHA-stimulated mononuclear cells and for the induction of proliferation by CFU-TL.

A wide variety of physical and chemical agents has been shown to have suppressive effects on T-lymphocyte colony formation (113,114,150–156). These include ionizing radiation (103), steroids (152,153), antimicrobial agents (154), cyclosporin A (155), lavamisole (156), and trace elements (F. D. Wilson, unpublished data). Abnormalities in T-lymphocyte colony formation have been observed in a variety of human diseases, including Fanconi's anemia (102), leukemia (103), and immune disorders (157,158).

In addition to the stimulation of T-lymphocyte colonies by nonspecific lectins, methods also exist for the growth of T lymphocytes in response to specific T-dependent antigens (104,109,110). Several groups have reported methods for the growth of T-lymphocyte colonies in semisolid culture systems in response to alloantigenic (mixed lymphocyte) stimulation (109,105,126). Wilson et al. (105), for example, reported a method for the growth of human T-lymphocyte colonies in response to alloantigenic stimulation of mononuclear cells from human peripheral blood. Colonies did not form to any major extent using autologous lymphocyte stimulation. Studies directly comparing the stimulation indexes achieved with standard mixed lymphocyte cultures utilizing [3]HTdr-incorporation to the colony-forming assay indicate that the cloning technique was far more sensitive for measuring allogeneic reactions than the [3]HTdr-incorporation technique and also produces less autologous (background) response. Thus, colony-forming techniques appear to provide a new and more sensitive method for the study of transplantation immunology.

A major advantage of the T-lymphocyte colony methods is that they permit identification and isolation of antigen-specific clones of T lymphocytes, which are present at very low levels. Stimulation of antigen-specific T-lymphocyte colony formation has been reported for mice (109,110) and humans (104,126). It is also possible to establish long-term, antigen-specific clonal lines by the use of TCGF (109,110).

Srendi et al. (109), for example, reported a method for cloning antigen-specific T lymphocytes from the lymph nodes of mice primed by a variety of hapten-carrier antigen combinations (i.e., PPD and DNP-OVA) that are known to be associated with delayed hypersensitivity (109,110). Such antigen-specific clones of T lymphocytes were initially isolated in semisolid cultures and were present at low cloning efficiencies (i.e., one colony per 2×10^5 lymphocytes plated), underlining the sensitivity to the technique. The antigen-specific clones were subsequently isolated and established by use of TCGF in continuous liquid-phase cultures at high cloning efficiency. For hapten-carrier-type antigens, the T cells were shown to be carrier specific in their recognition, but they were also capable of distinguishing the presence of the hapten.

In the previous section, methods for the growth of T-lymphocyte colonies from gradient-enriched mononuclear cell populations were described. In addition, Knox et al. (118) and Wilson et al. (112) reported a technique allowing for the growth of human (118) and canine (113) T-lymphocyte colonies directly in agarose without intervention of gradient-enrichment methods. The authors (112) proposed that the elimination of routine Ficoll-paque gradient used in lymphocyte isolation avoids potential problems of growth modulation due to elimination of nonlymphoid accessory cells and to the influences of gradients on selection for lymphocyte subpopulations. The technique was proposed to more closely approximate the *in vivo* mileu. Wilson et al. (112) and Knox et al. (118) compared mitogen-stimulated T-lymphocyte colony formation by whole blood with colonies produced from Ficoll-paque gradient-enriched mononuclear cells. Colony formation was also selectively stimulated by T-cell-dependent antigen PPD (using whole blood from a tuberculin-positive donor). Thus the technique would have potential application in the quantitation of clonal populations sensitized to specific antigenic determinants in addition to measuring polyclonal T-lymphocyte blastogenesis induced by nonspecific plant lectins.

Studies on radiation survival (103) indicated that the "whole blood" method was more sensitive than colony-forming techniques that used gradient-enriched mononuclear cells. Either colony method was more sensitive than standard ^{3}HTdr-incorporation techniques for the quantitation of radiation effects.

The "whole blood" colony technique was also applied to studies on patients with Fanconi's anemia (102). The cloning efficiencies and *in vitro* X-radiation dose-response characteristics of normal individuals and patients with Fanconi's anemia were compared using the whole blood T-lymphocyte colony technique and ^{3}HTdr-incorporation induced by PHA and ConA mitogens. The results (102) indicated Fanconi's anemia-associated abnormalities in PHA but not in ConA reactive sub-population of T lymphocytes. The selective PHA abnormality was reflected at two levels: an abnormally high cloning efficiency of the PHA subpopulation and a markedly increased susceptibility of the PHA subpopulation to the *in vitro* effects of ionizing radiation (102). The lymphocyte colony method was again found to be more sensitive than the ^{3}HTdr-incorporation technique. Additional studies using the whole blood T-lymphocyte colony technique have also demonstrated abnormalities in cloning efficiency and/or *in vitro* radiation survival characteristics in patients with a variety of hemopoietic disorders, including leukemias (104).

Methods are also available for the growth of B-lymphocyte colonies for humans (140–142) and experimental animals (9,129,139). Metcalf et al. (9) first reported the growth of B-lymphocyte colonies in semisolid agar in mice. The progenitor cells for B-lymphocyte colonies were termed CFU-BL (9). Mecaptoethanol was found to be necessary for the growth of B-lymphocyte colonies, and colony formation was enhanced by endotoxin and erythrocytes (133). The colony cells resembled immature lymphocytes and plasma cells by electron microscopy, possessed Fc receptors, and reacted with anti-μ-serum and anti-γ-serum. Evidence also indicated a clonogenic origin of the B-lymphocyte colonies (9). The clonal origin of CFU-BL was established by Lala and Johnson (131). CBA mice were injected with equal numbers of CBA and CBA T6/T6 hemopoietic cells. Cytogenetic analysis for the T6 marker of 7- to 15-day spleen colonies demonstrated that 90% were either exclusively T6 positive or T6 negative. Thus, CFU-BL are members of a hemopoietic clone derived from hemopoietic stem cells.

The influence of macrophage-derived factors on B-lymphocyte colony formation was studied by Kurland et al. (138,159). The effects of diffusable macrophage-derived factors (adherent peritoneal macrophages) on CFU-BL proliferation were studied using a double-layer culture system in mice (159). Macrophages incorporated within underlayers of spleen or lymph node cell cultures potentiated the number and size of B-lymphocyte colonies. However, when large numbers of macrophages were used, inhibition of colony formation was produced, and such inhibition was blocked by indomethacin, an inhibitor of prostaglandin synthesis.

Methods are also available for the growth of human B-cell colonies in semisolid culture systems (140,141). Roback and Whisler (140,141) described a method for the growth of human B lymphocytes from peripheral blood in response to stimulation by staphylococcal protein A. Those authors (140,141) further observed that T cells enhanced the B-lymphocyte colony formation.

Srendi et al. (142) recently reported on the long-term culture of normal human B lymphocytes isolated initially in semisolid culture. B-lymphocyte-enriched cells were first stimulated in suspension culture with mitogens and then B-lymphocyte colonies were produced using a double-layer agar culture system. Colony formation was T-cell-dependent and was optimum after presentation in suspension cultures containing PHA, PWM, or protein A. Individual colonies were picked from the semisolid cultures and subsequently propagated in suspension cultures by feeding them every 3 days with medium containing appropriately conditioned media prepared by stimulation of human peripheral blood mononuclear cells with PHA or PWA. The clonal lines could be propagated for up to 1 year. Thus, the technique allows for the long-term culture of normal (nontransformed) human B-lymphocyte clones.

CLONAL GROWTH OF PLURIPOTENT "STEM" OR PROGENITOR CELLS

Reference has already been made to techniques for the growth of primitive populations of committed progenitor cells for the granulocytic (36,37) and erythrocytic (85) differentiation pathways (CFU-D and BFU-E, respectively). Such "primitive" progenitors were initially thought to be intermediate in differentiation between pluripotent stem cells and unipotent progenitor cells (36,37,85). Recent studies have indicated that CFU-D (37) and BFU-E (85) are possibly more primitive than originally thought. In addition, the *in vitro* growth of pluripotent colony-forming cells exhibiting variable potential for pluripotentiality and self-replication has recently been described for experimental animals (17,160) and for humans (161,162). Further, studies have suggested that the progenitors of such mixed colonies (CFU-Mix) may represent the *in vitro* equivalent of *in vivo* pluripotent hemopoietic stem cells as measured by the spleen colony assay (CFU-S) (17,160–168).

Johnson and Metcalf (17) first observed that pokeweed mitogen spleen-cell-conditioned media stimulated the growth of both pure and mixed populations of erythroid colonies in 7-day agar cultures of mouse fetal liver cells. The progenitor cell for such mixed colonies was subsequently termed the colony-forming unit for mixed colonies or CFU-Mix. Such pure and mixed colonies were observed to form in the absence of detectable Epo (17). In addition to the erythrocytic elements, the most common hemopoietic elements observed in such mixed colonies were macrophages, neutrophils, eosinophils, and megakaryocytes—in that order (17). The colonal nature of such mixed colonies was confirmed by studies demonstrating their origin from single fetal liver cells isolated by micromanipulation (17).

Since the mixed colonies were clearly derived from pluripotent progenitor cells, the question of their potential relationship to pluripotent hemopoietic stem cells (CFU-S), as measured by the *in vivo* spleen-colony assay, was initially raised. The critical issue was the capacity of CFU-Mix for self-renewal in addition to the demonstrated pluripotentiality. To this aim Metcalf and Johnson (164) conducted recloning experiments and initially concluded that evidence for genuine self-replication was not present and that the CFU-Mix most likely represented a relatively differentiated but still multipotential stem cell.

Subsequent to the original description of CFU-Mix in mouse fetal liver (17), techniques have been reported for the growth of pluripotent mixed colonies in plasma on agar gels from a variety of tissues and species including humans (162,163). Similiar to colonies forming from fetal liver cells, the mixed colonies derived from adult hemopoietic tissues are composed of granulocytes, macrophages, erythrocytes, and megakaryocytes (163,164).

The presence of both T cells (163) and B cells (166) has been recently reported in mixed colonies. The clonal origin of such mixed colonies also has been reported (17,160). The exact composition of mixed colonies forming from the pluripotent progenitors depends on the addition of specific growth stimulants [pokeweed mitogen spleen-cell-conditioned media, PHA-induced leukocyte-conditioned medium (PHA-LCM), Epo, or PHA; refs. 17,160–168] and appears to be a two-step process. For example, PHA-LCM appears to stimulate both proliferation of the pluripotent progenitor cells (CFU-Mix) and differentiation of CFU-Mix into the various committed unipotent progenitor cells. Once the various committed progenitors are formed, they are subsequently stimulated to proliferate and differentiate by various specific growth factors. For example, mixed erythroid colonies occur if Epo is added at day 4 or day 5 of culture, but do not form if Epo is omitted (160). In addition to stimulation of CFU-Mix proliferation, PHA-LCM also provide for a source of the specific growth promotor of granulocyte-macrophage committed progenitors (GM-CSF) (160). The development of T cells in mixed colonies occurs in response to either T-cell growth factor or PHA (164).

More recently Ogawa et al. (167) and Nakahata and Ogawa (168) reported on a class of hemopoietic progenitors in mouse and human bone marrow that appeared to be more primitive than CFU-Mix. Such progenitors produced a small colony consisting of undifferentiated blast cells even after prolonged incubation in the presence of lectin-stimulated LCM (167). Such blast (stem) cell colonies were demonstrated by recloning experiments to be capable of self-replication and were capable of generating large numbers of secondary GEMM colonies. In contrast, GEMM colonies upon replicating failed to produce blast cell colonies and only small numbers of GEMM colonies.

METHODS FOR THE CONTINUOUS GROWTH OF PLURIPOTENT HEMOPOIETIC STEM CELLS *IN VIVO*

In addition to the techniques for the short-term growth of pluripotent hemopoietic progenitors in semisolid culture systems, methods are also available for the long-term growth of pluripotent hemopoietic stem cells using liquid-phase culture systems (23,169–174). Dexter et al. (169) were the first to describe the long-term maintenance of pluripotent hemopoietic stem cells (CFU-S) in suspension cultures of mouse bone marrow. In the original method (169), mouse bone marrow cells were grown in tissue culture medium containing horse serum. The cultures were fed weekly by removing half the growth medium and adding fresh medium. It was observed that over a 2- to 3-week period, an adherent layer composed of cells representative of marrow stromal elements was formed (169,170). When fully developed, adherent cells are reinoculated with additional syngeneic, allogeneic, or semiallogeneic marrow cells. Maintenance of CFU-S and committed progenitors (CFU-GM, BFU-E, CFU-Meg) was observed for several months (23,169–174). The presence of the adherent layer composed of macrophages, epithelioid cells, fibroblasts, and fat cells was found to be an absolute requirement for the long-term culture of stem cells (169).

The demonstration that adherent cells forming in cultures of bone marrow provide a microenvironment absolutely necessary for the long-term maintenance of stem and progenitor cells *in vitro* has provided an exciting stimulus to investigations of microenvironmental regulation of hemopoiesis. Although originally described for mice (169), long-term culture systems have now been developed for several specimen including humans (29). In addition to pluripotent hemopoietic stem cells (CFU-S), the adherent layers support growth of a variety of committed stem cells, including CFU-GM (169), BFU-E (171), and magakaryocyte progenitors (172).

A relationship of the *in vitro* adherent cells to hemopoietic microenvironment was further suggested by the demonstration that the bone marrow adherent cells obtained from mice with genetic stomal-associated anemia (Sl/Sl^d anemia) were defective in their capacity to support stem cell proliferation in long-term cultures (23). Further, the defect could be "cured" by the addition of adherent cells from normal donors (23). It should be mentioned, however, that the long-term growth of hemopoietic stem cells in the absence of adherent layers has recently been reported for hamster bone marrow and spleen cells (174).

The liquid-culture system provides a unique opportunity for studying a range of problems associated with hemopoietic cellular proliferation, differentiation, and maturation. Foremost of these is the role of marrow-supportive stroma in the determination of stem cell proliferation. Further, the long-term culture system provides a model for the *in vitro* effects produced by chronic myelotoxicity.

METHODS FOR THE GROWTH OF BONE MARROW FIBROBLAST COLONIES

There are two major reasons for studying bone marrow fibroblast populations and their progenitors. The first is evidence suggesting that bone marrow stroma (and specifically fibroblast or adventitial reticular cells) are involved in the microenvironmental regulation of hemopoiesis (10,11,19–24,169–193). The second reason is that bone marrow fibroblasts are major pathological components of various hemopoietic disorders associated with the development of myelofibrosis (19,194,195). Also, studies have suggested that abnormalities in marrow fibroblast may be associated with the development of some forms of aplastic anemia (182,183,203) and leukemia (195,201,204). Reference has already been made to the absolute requirement of fibroblasts (and other adherent cells) for the long-term growth of stem and progenitor cells in suspension cultures (23,30,169–174,176) and to abnormalities in adherent cells in stromal-based genetic (Sl/Sl^d) anemia in mice (23). In addition, extensive *in vivo* evidence for "microenvironmental" regulatory effects of fibroblasts has been reported (10,11,19–24,175–177,179–182,184,186).

Numerous techniques for the clonal growth of bone marrow fibroblasts in experimental animals and humans have been reported (22–24,178,185,187–193,195–213). Reports as early as those published by Maximow (192) have described the growth of fibroblastic elements from bone marrow and other hemopoietic tissues using a variety of culture systems. However, until relatively recently, the true origin, functional nature, and differentiation capacities of such *in vitro* fibroblastic populations were not known. In the early 1970s, Friedenstein et al. (22) described the growth of surface-adherent fibroblastic colonies in liquid-phase culture systems of guinea pig and mouse bone marrow. Those authors demonstrated that the fibroblastic elements, when harvested and transplanted into diffusion chambers subsequently implanted into the peritoneal cavity of animal hosts, gave rise *in vivo* to stromal elements associated with the production of reticular fibers, collagen, and bone. Briefly, the technique employed for the growth of fibroblast colonies by those authors (22) involved the inoculation of single-cell preparations of spleen or bone marrow into tissue culture vessels containing 80% tissue culture media and 20% bovine serum. The media were completely replaced following 24-hour incubation at 37°. On subsequent incubation the formation of discrete surface-adherent colonies of fibroblasts was observed and thus the number of fibroblast progenitors (CFU-F) could be quantitated. Studies have also demonstrated a clonogenic origin of the fibroblast colonies (22,191).

Subsequently, a variety of methods for the growth of CFU-F including for humans has been reported (22–24,178,185,187–213), as have numerous studies on the characterization of CFU-F and on the fibroblastic progenitors (22,178,185,187,188–213).

In an elegant extension of his earlier work on fibroblasts, Friedenstein et al. (22) further demonstrated not only that bone marrow or splenic isolates of fibroblasts contained stromal differentiation capacity when implanted *in vivo*, but also that microenvironmental information for the differentiation of hemopoietic stem cells was transmitted by the fibroblast (3). In those studies, adherent stromal cells (fibroblasts) were first isolated in tissue cultures prepared from the spleen and bone marrow of rabbits (3). Following 4 to 10 days' growth *in vitro*, the fibroblasts were harvested by trypsinization and were subsequently transplanted as a pellet under the renal capsule or subcutaneously into recipient mice. In agreement with the previous studies, it was found that the implanted marrow-derived fibroblast isolates resulted in the formation of bone ossicles containing hemopoietic elements within the medullary cavities that formed. In contrast, isolated spleen fibroblasts did not form bone, but gave rise only to reticular tissue and supported lymphoid rather than myeloid elements.

The authors concluded (22) that stromal progenitors, as indicated by the growth of fibroblast colonies *in vitro*, contain information for the transfer of the microenvironment typical of the parent tissue (spleen or marrow) from which the isolates were originally derived. Patt et al. (180) reached similar results for the *in vivo* differentiation and support capacity of bone marrow stromal isolates obtained for red and yellow marrow sites.

The effects of various myelotoxic agents on bone marrow CFU-F have been reported (24,185,213), and abnormalities in marrow fibroblasts have been observed in various hemopoietic disorders in humans (195,201,203,207,208,209) and experimental animals (196,199,200,210,211).

SUMMARY

The lymphohemopoietic system is uniquely sensitive to a wide variety of toxic agents. Such susceptibility to toxins fundamentally relates to the physiological demands for rapid and extensive cell renewal. Thus, populations of lymphohemopoietic stem and progenitor cells that are capable of self-renewal, proliferation, and diverse differentiation capacity must exist to meet continual cellular demands. These populations of stem and progenitor cells are especially sensitive to toxic agents, particularly chemicals producing DNA-inhibitory effects. A wide variety of *in vitro* techniques exist for the clonogenic growth of lympho-myeloid stem and progenitor cells in semisolid culture systems. Such methods are available for studies on humans and experimental animals. The functional nature of the clonogenic population that develops in culture is dependent on the presence of specific growth factors. Culture systems are available for the growth of pluripotent stem cells, "stromal" cells, and a varitey of committed progenitor cells (neutrophil, eosinophil, monocyte, macrophage, erythrocyte, megakaryocyte, B lymphocytes, and T lymphocytes). Techniques are also available for the long-term growth of pluripotent hemopoietic stem cells. In this chapter the various techniques for the clonal growth of lymphohemopoietic stem and progenitor cells were reviewed with particular emphasis on their application to studies on myelotoxicity and immunotoxicity.

REFERENCES

1. Metcalf, D. (1977): In: *Hemopoietic Colonies: In Vitro Cloning of Normal and Leukemic Cells*, edited by G. P. Rentchnick, Springer-Verlag, Berlin.
2. Metcalf, D., and Moore, M. A. S. (1971): *Haemopoietic Cells*. North-Holland, Amsterdam and London.
3. Till, J. E., and McCulloch, E. A. (1961): A direct measurement of the radiation sensitivity of normal mouse bone marrow cells. *Radiat. Res.*, 14:213–222.
4. Iscove, N. N. (1978): Erythropoietin-independent stimulation of early erythropoiesis in adult marrow cultures by conditioned media from lectin-stimulated mouse spleen cells. *In: Hematopoietic Cell Differentiation*, edited by D. W. Golde, M. J. Clinic, and C. F. Fox, pp. 37–52. Academic Press, New York.
5. Stephenson, J. R., Axelrad, A. A., McLeod, D. L., and Shreeve, M. M. (1971): Induction of colonies of hemoglobin synthesizing cells by erythropoietin in vitro. *Proc. Natl. Acad. Sci. USA*, 68:1542–1549.
6. Metcalf, D. (1973): Regulation of granulocyte and monocyte-macrophage proliferation by colony stimulating factor (CSF): A review. *Exp. Hematol.*, 1:185–201.

7. Nakeff, A., and Daniels-McQueen, S. (1976): In vitro colony assay for a new class of megakaryocyte precursor: Colony-forming unit, megakaryocyte (CFU-M). *Proc. Soc. Exp. Biol. Med.*, 151:587–594.
8. Srendi B., Kalechman, Y., Michlin, H., and Rosenszain, L. A. (1976): Development of colonies in vitro of mitogen-stimulated mouse T-lymphocytes. *Nature*, 259:130–132.
9. Metcalf, D., Nossal, G. J. V., Warner, W. L., Miller, J. F. A. P., Mendel, T. E., Layton, J. E., and Guttman, G. A. (1975): Growth of B-lymphocyte colonies in vitro. *J. Exp. Med.*, 142:1534–1548.
10. Cline, M. J., and Golde, D. W. (1979): Cellular interactions in hematopoiesis. *Nature*, 277:177–181.
11. Bessis, M. C., and Brenton-Gorius (1962): Iron metabolism in the bone marrow as seen by electron microscopy: A critical review. *Blood*, 19:635–663.
12. Kurland, J. I., Kincade, P. W., Moore, M. A. S. (1977): Regulation of B-lymphocyte clonal proliferation by stimulatory and inhibitory macrophage-derived factors. *J. Exp. Med.*, 146:1420–1435.
13. Kurland, J. I., and Moore, M. A. S. (1977): Modulation of hemopoiesis by prostaglandins. *Exp. Hematol.*, 5:257–264.
14. Kurland, J. I. (1978): The mononuclear phagocyte and its regulatory interactions in hemopoiesis. *In: Experimental Hematology Today*, edited by S. J. Baum, and G. D. Ledney, pp. 47–60. Springer-Verlag, New York.
15. Chen, S. Y., Renold, H. G., Westbrook, C. A., Gwopman, J. E., Lusis, A. J., Golde, D. W. (1983): Human lymphokines and hematopoiesis. *J. Cell. Biochem.*, *[Suppl.]* 713:5.
16. Cline, M. J., and Golde, D. W. (1974): Production of colony-stimulating activity by human lymphocytes. *Nature*, 248:703–704.
17. Johnson, G. R., and Metcalf, D. (1977): Pure and mixed erythroid colony formation in vitro stimulated by spleen conditioned medium with no detectable erythropoietin. *Proc. Natl. Acad. Sci. U.S.A.*, 74:3879–3885.
18. Castro-Malaspina, H., and Moore, M. A. S. (1982): Pathophysiological mechanisms operating in the development of myelofibrosis: Role of myeloproliferative disorders. *Nouv. Rev. Fr. Hematol.*, 24:221–226.
19. Trentin, J. J. (1977): Determination of bone marrow stem cell differentiation by stromal hemopoietic inductive microenvironments (HIM). *Am. J. Pathol.*, 65:621–628.
20. Tavassoli, M. (1975): Studies on hemopoietic microenvironments. *Exp. Hematol.*, 3:213–226.
21. Wolf, N. S., and Trentin, J. J. (1968): Hemopoietic colony studies. V. Effect of hemopoietic organ stroma on differentiation of pluripotent stem cells. *J. Exp. Med.*, 127:205–214.
22. Friedenstein, A. J., Chailakhyan, R. K., Lastinik, N. V., Panasyuk, N. V., Panasyuk, A. F., and Keliss-Borok, I. V. (1974): Stromal cells responsible for transferring the microenvironment of the hemopoietic tissues. *Transplantation*, 17:331–340.
23. Dexter, T. M., and Moore, M. A. S. (1977): In vitro duplication and "cure" of haemopoietic defects in genetically anaemic mice. *Nature*, 269:412–414.
24. Wilson, F. D., O'Grady, L., McNeil, C. J., and Monn, S. L. (1974): The formation of bone marrow derived fibroblastic plaques in vitro: Preliminary results contrasting these populations to CFU-C. *Exp. Hematol.*, 2:343–353.
25. Van Bekkum, D. W., VanNoord, M. J., Maat, B., and Dicke, K. A. (1971): Attempts at identification of hemopoietic stem cells in mouse. *Blood*, 38:547–559.
26. Norwell, P. C., Hersch, B. E., Fox, B. H., and Wilson, D. B. (1970): Evidence for the existence of multipotential lympho-hematopoietic stem cells in the adult rat. *J. Cell Physiol.*, 75:151–158.
27. Lajtha, L. G., Pozzi, L. V., Schofield, R., and Fox, M. (1969): Kinetics and properties of haemopoietic stem cells. *Cell. Tissue. Kinet.*, 2:39–43.
28. Calvo, W., Fliedner, T. M., Herbst, E., Hugl, E., and Bruch, C. (1976): Regeneration of blood-forming organs after autologous leukocyte transfusion in lethally irradiated dogs. II. Distribution and cellularity of the marrow in irradiated and transfused animals. *Blood*, 47:593–601.
29. Moore, M. A. S., Broxmeyer, H. E., Sheridan, A. P. C., Meyers, P. A., Jacobsen, N., and Whinchester, R. J. (1980): Continuous human bone marrow culture: Ia antigen characterization of probable pluripotent stem cells. *Blood*, 55:682–690.
30. Dexter, T. M., Allen, T. D., Lajtha, L. G., Schofield, R., and Lord, B. I. (1973): Stimulation of differentiation of haemopoietic cells in vitro. *J. Cell. Physiol.*, 82:461–473.
31. Dexter, T. M., Allen, T. D., and Lajtha, L. G. (1977): Conditions controlling the proliferation of haemopoietic stem cells in vitro. *J. Cell. Physiol.*, 191:335–343.

32. Bradley, T. R., and Metcalf, D. (1966): The growth of mouse bone marrow cells in vitro. *Aust. J. Exp. Biol. Med. Sci.*, 44:286–293.
33. Pluznik, D. H., and Sachs, L. (1966): The induction of clones of normal mast cells by a substance from conditioned medium. *Exp. Cell. Res.*, 43:553–563.
34. Nakeff, A., Dicke, K. A., and VanNoord, M. J. (1974): Megakaryocytes in agar cultures of mouse bone marrow. *Ser. Haematol.*, 8:275–289.
35. Metcalf, D., Parker, J., Chester, H. M., and Kincade, P. W. Formation of eosinophil-like granulocyte colonies by mouse bone marrow cells in vitro. *J. Cell Physiol.*, 84:275–289.
36. Boyum, A., and Borgstrom, R. (1970): The concentration of granulocytic stem cells in mouse bone marrow determined with diffusion chamber technique. *Scand. J. Haematol.* 7:294–303.
37. Jacobsen, N., Broxmeyer, H. E., Grossbard, E., and Moore, M. .A. S. (1979): Colony-forming units in diffusion chamber (CPU-d) and colony-forming units in agar culture (CFU-C) obtained from normal human bone marrow: A possible parent-progeny relationship. *Cell Tissue Kinet.* 12:213–219.
38. Burgess, A. W., Wilson, E. M. A., and Metcalf, D. (1977): Stimulation by human placental conditioned medium of hemopoietic colony formation by human marrow cells. *Blood*, 49:573–583.
39. Lusis, A. J., Quon, D. H., and Bolde, D. W. (1981): Purification and characterization of a T-lymphocyte-derived granulocyte-macrophage colony-stimulating factor. *Blood*, 57:13–21.
40. DiPersio, J. F., Brennan, J. K., Lichtman, M. A., and Speiser, B. L. (1978): Human cell lines that elaborate colony-stimulating activity for the marrow cells of man and other species. *Blood*, 51:507–519.
41. Ruscetti, F. W., Chev, J. V., and Gallo, R. C. (1978): Human trophoblasts: cellular source of colony-stimulating activity in placental tissue. *Blood*, 59:86–93.
42. Burgess, A. W., and Metcalf, D. (1980): The nature and action of granulocyte-macrophage colony stimulating factors. *Blood*, 56:947–958.
43. Nicole, N. A., Metcalf, D., Johnson, G. R., and Burgess, A. W. (1979): Separation of functionally distinct human granulocyte-macrophage colony stimulating factors, *Blood*, 54:614–627.
44. Wu, M. C., Miller, A. W., and Yunis, A. A. (1981): Immunological and functional differences between human type I and II colony-stimulating factors. *J. Clin. Invest.*, 67:1588–1591.
45. Pigoli, G., Waheed, A., and Shadduck, R. K. (1982): Observations on the binding and interaction of radioiodinated colony-stimulating factors with murine bone marrow cells in vitro. *Blood*, 59:408–413.
46. Guilbert, L. J., and Stanley, E. R. (1980): Specific interaction of murine colony stimulating factor with mononuclear phagocytic cells. *J. Cell. Biol.*, 85:153–164.
47. Bryne, P. V., Guilbert, L. J., and Stanley, R. (1981): Distribution of cells bearing receptors for colony-stimulating factor (CSF-1) in murine tissues. *J. Cell. Biol.*, 91:848–853.
48. Pike, P. V., and Robinson, W. A. (1980): Human bone marrow colony growth in agar-gel. *J. Cell Physiol.*, 76:77–84.
49. Lajtha, L. G., Pozzi, L. Y., Schofield, R., and Fox, M. (1969): Kinetic properties of haemopoietic stem cells. *Cell Tissue Kinet.*, 2:39–43.
50. Haskill, T. A., McNeill, T. A., and Moore, M. A. S. (1970): Density distribution analysis of in vivo and in vitro colony forming cells in bone marrow. *J. Cell Physiol.*, 75:167–179.
51. Sutherland, D. J. A., Till, J. E., and McCulloch, E. A. (1970): A kinetic study of the genetic control of hemopoietic progenitor cells assayed in culture and in vivo. *J. Cell. Physiol.*, 75:89–96.
52. Chan, M. G., and Schooley, J. C. (1970): Recovery of proliferative capacity of agar colony-forming cells and spleen colony-forming cells following ionizing radiation or vinblastine. *J. Cell. Physiol.*, 75:89–96.
53. Rickard, K. A., Shadduck, R. K., Howard, D. E., and Stohlman, F., Jr. (1970): A differential effect of hydroxyurea on hematopoietic stem cell colonies in vitro and in vivo. *Proc. Soc. Exp. Biol. Med.*, 134:152–156.
54. Metcalf, D. (1983): Regulation of self-replication in normal and leukemic stem cells. *J. Cell Biochem.*, [Suppl.] 7B:4.
55. Pavan, M., and Sacks, L. (1968): The continued requirement for inducer for the development of macrophage and granulocyte colonies. *J. Cell Physiol.*, 72:247–253.
56. Metcalf, D., and Foster, R., Jr. (1967): Behavior on transfer of serum stimulated bone marrow colonies. *Proc. Soc. Exp. Biol. Med.*, 126:758–765.

57. Burgess, A. W., and Metcalf, D. (1977): The effect of colony stimulating factor on the synthesis of ribonucleic acid by mouse bone marrow cells in vitro, *J. Cell Physiol.*, 96:471–479.

58. Wing, E. J., Waheed, A., Shadduck, A. R. K., Nagle, L. S., and Stephensen, B. A. (1982): Effect of colony stimulating factor on murine macrophages: Induction of antitumor acitivity, *J. Clin. Invest.*, 69:270–276.

59. Stanley, E. R., and Guilbert, L. J. (1981): Methods for the purification, assay, characterization and target cell binding of colony stimulating factor (CSF-1) *J. Immunol. Methods*, 42:253–257.

60. Tushinski, R. J., Oliver, I. T., Guilbert, L. J., Tyham, P. W., Wanner, J. R., and Stanley, E. R. (1982): *Cell*, 28:71–83.

61. Das, S. K., Stanley, E. R., Guilbert, L. J., and Forman, L. W. (1981): Human colony-stimulating factor (CSF-1) radioimmunoassay: Resolution of three subclasses of human colony stimulating factors. *Blood*, 58:630–641.

62. Guilbert, L. J., and Stanley, E. R. (1980): Specific interaction of murine colony-stimulating factor with mononuclear phagocytic cells. *J. Cell Biol.*, 85:153–161.

63. Bryne, P. V., Guilbert, L. J., and Stanley, E. R. (1981): Distribution of cells bearing receptors for a colony-stimulation factor (CSF-1) in murine tissues. *J. Cell Biol.*, 91:848–853.

64. Moore, M. A. S., and Pelus, L. M. (1983): Regulation of proliferation and differentiation of normal and leukemic CFU-GM. *J. Cell. Biochem. [Suppl.]* 7B:6.

65. Barranco, S. C., and Novak, J. F. (1974): Survival responses of dividing and non-dividing mammalian cells after treatment with hydroxyurea, arabinosylcytosine or adriamycin. *Cancer Res.*, 34:1616–1618.

66. Domenil, D., Sainteny, F., and Frindel, E. (1979): Some effects of chemotherapeutic drugs on bone marrow stem cells. *Cancer Chemother. Pharmacol.*, 2:197–204.

67. Radley, J. M., and Sevrfield, S. (1979): Effect of 5-flurouracil on mouse bone marrow. *Br. J. Haematol.*, 43:341–349.

68. Yunis, A. A., and Gross, M. A. (1975): Drug-induced inhibition of myeloid colony growth: protective effect of colony stimulating factor. *J. Lab. Clin. Med.*, 86:499–504.

69. Yunis, A. A., and Adamson, J. W. (1977): Differential in vitro sensitivity of marrow erythroid and granulocyte colony forming units to chloramphenicol. *Am. J. Hematol.*, 2:355–363.

70. Pigoli, S., Mangoni, L., Caramitti, C., Degliantoni, G., and Rozzoli, V. (1983): Inhibition of murine CFU-C by vindesine: Restoration of colony growth by colony stimulating factor. *Int. J. Cell. Colony.*, 1:143–147.

71. Gordon, M. Y., Blackett, N. M., and Douglas, I. D. C. (1975): Colony formation by human haemopoietic precursor cells cultured in semisolid agar diffusion chambers. *Br. J. Haematol.*, 31:103–111.

72. Gordon, M. Y. (1976): Changes in human bone marrow colony-forming cells following chemotherapy using agar diffusion-chamber technique. *In: Experimental Hematology Today*, edited by S. J. Baum, and G. D. Ledney, p. 233, Springer-Varlag, New York.

73. Gordon, M. Y., and Blackett, N. M. (1975): Stimulation of granulocyte colony formation in agar diffusion chambers implanted in cyclophosphamide pretreated mice. *Br. J. Cancer*, 32:51–57.

74. Gordon, M. Y., and Blackett, N. M. (1976): The sensitivity of human and murine haemopoietic precursor cells exposed to cytotoxic drugs in an in vivo culture system. *Cancer Res.*, 36:2822–2826.

75. Niskamen, E. (1983): Parent-progeny relationship between murine CFU-S and CFU-D *J. Cellular Biochem.*, *[Suppl.]* 7B:25.

76. Jacobson, L. D., Gurney, C. W., Plzak, L., and Fried, W. (1957): Studies on erythropoiesis. IV. Reticulocyte response of hypophysectomized and polycythemic/rodents to erythropoietin. *Proc. Soc. Exp. Biol. Med.*, 94:243–247.

77. Axelrad, A. A., McLeod, D. L., Shreeve, M. M., and Heath, D. S. (1974): Properties of cells that produce erythrocytic colonies in vitro. *In: Hemopoiesis in Culture*, edited by W. Robinson, U.S. Government Printing Office, Washington, D.C.

78. Axelrad, A. A., McLeod, D. L., Shreeve, M. M., and Heath, D. S. (1973): Properties of cells that produce erythrocytic colonies in plasma culture. *In Proceedings of the Second International Workshop on Hemopoiesis in Culture*, edited by W. A. Robinson, pp. 79–86. Grune and Stratton, New York.

79. Iscove, N. N., and Sieber, R. (1975): Macroscopic erythroid colony formation in culture of mouse bone marrow cells. *Exp. Hematol.*, 3:32–43.

80. Heath, D. S., Axelrad, A. A., McLeod, D. L., and Shreeve, M. M. (1976): Separation of eryth-

ropoietin-responsible progenitors BFU-E and CFU-E in mouse bone marrow by unit gravity sedimentation. *Blood*, 47:777–792.
81. Iscove, N. N., Sieber, F., and Winterhalter, K. H. (1974): Erythroid colony formation in cultures of mouse and human bone marrow: Analysis of the requirement for erythropoietin by gel filtration and affinity chromatography on agarose-concanavalin A. *J. Cell. Physiol.*, 83:309–320.
82. Gregory, D. J., Tepperman, A. D., McCulloch, E. A., and Till, J. E. (1973): Erythropoietic progenitor cells capable of colony formation in culture: Response of normal and genetically anemic W/W^v mice to manipulation of the erythron. *J. Cell Physiol.*, 91:411–421.
83. Cooper, M. C., Levy, J., Cantor, L. N., Marks, P. A., and Rifkind, R. A. (1974): The effect of erythropoietin on colonial growth of erythroid precursor cells in vitro. *Proc. Natl. Acad. Sci. USA*, 71:1677–1684.
84. Aye, M. T. (1977): Erythroid colony formation in cultures of human marrow: Effects of leukocyte conditioned medium. *Blood*, 91:69.
85. Wagemaker, G. (1978): Induction of erythropoietin responsiveness in vitro. *In: Hematopoietic Cell Differentiation*, edited by D. W. Golde, M. J. Cline, and C. F. Fox, pp. 109–118. Academic Press, New York.
86. Wagemaker, G., Ober-Kieftenburg, V. E., Browner, A., and Peters-Slough, M. F. (1976): Some characteristics of in vitro erythroid colony and burst-forming units. *In: Experimental Hematology Today*, edited by S. J. Baum, and G. D. Ledney, p. 103, Springer-Verlag, New York.
87. Wagemaker, G., and Peters, M. F. (1978): *Cell Tissue Kinet.*, 11:43–48.
88. McLeod, D. L., Shreeve, M. M., and Axelrod, A. A. (1976): Induction of megakaryocyte colonies with platelet formation in vitro. *Nature (Lond.)*, 261:492–494.
89. Nakeff, A., Dicke, K. A., and VanNoord, M. J. (1975): Megakaryocytes in agar cultures of mouse marrow. *Ser. Hematol.*, 8:4–15.
90. Metcalf, D., MacDonald, H. R., Odartchenko, N., and Sordat, B. (1975): Growth of mouse megakaryocyte colonies in vitro. *Proc. Natl. Acad. Sci. USA*, 72:744–756.
91. Nakeff, A. (1977): *In: Experimental Hematology Today*, edited by S. J. Baum, and G. D. Ledney, pp. 111–123. Springer-Verlag, New York.
92. Nakeff, A., and Bryan, J. E. (1978): Megakaryocyte proliferation and its regulation as revealed by CFU-M analysis. *In: Hematopoietic Cell Differentiation*, edited by D. W. Golde, M. J. Cline, D. Metcalf, and C. F. Fox, pp. 241–259, Academic Press, New York.
93. Nakeff, A., and Dicke, K. A. (1976): Stem cell differentiation into megakaryocytes from mouse bone marrow cultured with the thin layer technique. *Exp. Hematol.* 22:58–64.
94. Nakeff, A., and Floeh, D. P. (1976): Seperation of megakaryocytes from mouse bone marrow by density gradient centrifugation. *Blood*, 48:133–138.
95. Nakeff, A. (1976): Colony-forming unit megakaryocyte (CFU-M): Its use in elucidating the kinetics and humoral control of the megakaryocytic committed progenitor cell compartment. *In: Experimental Hematology Today*, edited by S. J. Baum, and G. D. Ledney, pp. 111–123, Springer-Verlag, New York.
96. Odell, T. T., Jr. (1974): Megakaryocytopoiesis and its response to stimulation and suppression. *In: Platelets: Production, Function, Transfusion and Storage*, edited by Baldini and S. Ebbe, p. 11, Grune and Stratton, New York.
97. Bernstein, S. E., Russell, E. S., and Keighley, G. (1968): Two hereditary mouse anemias (S1/S1^d and W/W^v) deficiantion in response to erythropoietin. *Ann. NY Acad. Sci.*, 149:475–483.
98. Ebbe, S., Phalen, E., and Stohlman, F., Jr. (1973): Abnormalities of megakaryocytes in W/W^v mice. *Blood*, 42:857–864.
99. Ebbe, S., Phalen, E., and Stohlman, F., Jr. (1973): Abnormalities of megakaryocytes in S1/S1^d mice. *Blood*, 42:865–871.
100. Mazur, E. M., deAlarcon, P., South, K., and Miceli, L. (1983): Evidence that human megakaryocytopoiesis is controlled in vivo by a humoral factor. *J. Cell Biochem., [Suppl.]* 7B:28.
101. Stahn, R., Fabricius, H. A., and Hartleitnew, W. (1978): Suppression of human T-cell colony formation during pregnancy. *Nature*, 276:831–832.
102. Knox, S. J., Wilson, F. D., Greenberg, B. R., Shifrine, M., Rosenblatt, L. S., Reeves, J. D., and Misra, H. (1981): Increased radiosensitivity of subpopulations of T-lymphocyte progenitors from patients with Fanconi's anemia. *Blood*, 57:1043–1048.
103. Knox, S. J., Shifrine, M., and Rosenblatt, L. S. (1982): Assessment of the in vitro radiosensitivity of human peripheral blood lymphocytes. *Radiat. Res.*, 89:575–589.
104. Knox, S. J., Wilson, F. D., Shifrine, M., Greenberg, B. R., Dyck, J. A., and Rosenblatt, L. S.

(1980): Growth of human and canine T-lymphocyte colonies from whole blood: Applications of lymphocyte colony-forming techniques. *In: Experimental Hematology Today*, edited by S. J. Baum and G. D. Ledney, pp. 203–211. Springer-Verlag, New York.

105. Wilson, F. D., Whaley, C. B., Shifrine, M., Dyck, J. A., Carbonell, A. R., and Hinds, D. (1980): The formation of human lymphocyte colonies in semisolid cultures in response to allogeneic mixed-lymphocyte stimulation. *Exp. Hematol.*, 8:802–815.

106. Rozenszain, L. A., Shoham, D., and Kalechman, L. A. (1976): Development of colonies in vitro of mitogen-stimulated mouse T-lymphocytes. *Nature*, 259:130–132.

107. Rosenberg, S. A., Spiess, P. J., and Schwarz, S., (1980): In vitro growth of murine T cells. *Cell. Immunol.*, 54:293–306.

108. Ching, L-M., and Miller, R. G. (1980): Characterization of in vitro T-lymphocyte colonies from normal mouse spleen cells: Colonies containing cytotoxic lymphocyte precursors. *J. Immunol.*, 124:696–701.

109. Srendi, B., Tse, H. Y., Chen, C., and Schwartz, R. H. (1981): Antigen-specific clones of proliferating T-lymphocytes I. Methodology, specificity, and MHC restriction. *J. Immunol.*, 126:341–347.

110. Srendi, B., Matis, L. A., Lerner, E. A., Paul, W. E., and Schwartz, R. H. (1981): Antigen-specific T-cell clones restricted to unique F_1 major histocompatibility complex determinants. Inhibition of proliferation with a monoclonal anti-Ia antibody. *J. Exp. Med.*, 153:677–693.

111. Wilson, F. D., Shifrine, M., Gershwin, M. E., Spangler, W., and Dyck, J. (1978): Growth of canine T-lymphocyte colonies in vitro. *Exp. Hematol.*, 6:549–557.

112. Wilson, F. D., Dyck, J. A., Knox, S. J., and Shifrine, M. (1980): A "whole blood" technique for the quantitation of canine "T-lymphocyte" progenitors using a semisolid culture system. *Exp. Hematol.*, 8:1031–1039.

113. Rozenszain, L. A., Shoham, D., and Kalechman, I. (1975): Clonal proliferation of PHA-stimulated human lymphocytes in soft agar culture. *Immunology*, 29:1041–1055.

114. Fibach, E., Gerassi, E., and Sachs, L. (1976): Induction of colony formation in vitro by human lymphocytes. *Nature*, 259:127–129.

115. Pistoria, V., Ghio, R., Canonica, G. W., Colombatti, M., and Moretta, L. (1981): Comparison of the colony-forming capacity of human T-lymphocyte sub-populations. *Clin. Immunol. Immuopath.*, 21:289–294.

116. Ulner, A. J., and Flad, H-D. (1979): One stage stimulation of human T-lymphocyte colony-forming units (TL-CFU) in a micro agar culture in glass capillaries. *Immunology*, 38:393–400.

117. Gelfand, E. W., Lee, J. W. W., Bosch, H-M., and Price, G. B. (1981): Human T cell colony formation in microculture: Analysis of growth requirements and functional activities. *J. Immunol.*, 126:1134–1139.

118. Knox, S. J., Shifrine, M., Wilson, F. D., and Rosenblatt, L. S. (1981): The selective growth of human T-lymphocyte colonies from whole blood in a semisolid culture system. *Exp. Hematol.*, 9:926–937.

119. Triebel, F., Robinson, W. A., Hayward, A. R., and Goube de LaForest, P. (1981): Characterization of the lymphocyte colony-forming cells and evidence for the acquisition of T cell markers in the absence of the thymic microenvironmental in man. *J. Immunol.*, 126:2020–2023.

120. Triebel, F., Robinson, W. A., Hayward, A. R., and Goube de Laforest, P. (1981): Existence of a pool of T-lymphocyte colony-forming cells (T-CFC) in human bone marrow and their place in the differentiation of the T-lymphocyte lineage. *Blood*, 58:911–915.

121. Klein, B., Caraux, J., Thomas, P., and Goube de LaForest, P. (1982): Nature and mechanisms of action of co-operating cells controlling T-colony formation. *Immunology*, 45:265–271.

122. Sachs, L. (1978): Control of cloning of normal human T-lymphocytes by transferring albumin and different lectins. *Clin. Exp. Immunol.*, 33:495–498.

123. Claesson, M. H., Rodger, M. B., Johnson, G. R., Whittingham, S., and Metcalf, D. (1977): Colony formation by human T-lymphocytes in agar medium. *Clin. Exp. Immunol.*, 28:526–531.

124. Shen, J., Wilson, F., Shifrine, M., and Gershwin, M. E. (1977): Select growth of human T-lymphocytes in single phase semisolid culture, *J. Immunol.*, 119:1299–1305.

125. Mercola, K., and Cline, M. J. (1979): A new clonogenic technique for human mitogen-responsive cells. *J. Immunol.*, 123:1721–1725.

126. Kornbluth, J., and Dupont, B. (1980): Colony and functional characterization of primary alloreactive human T-lymphocytes. *J. Exp. Med.*, 152:164–171.

127. Kornbluth, J., Silver, D. M., and Dupont, B. (1981): Cloning and characterization of primary alloreactive human T-lymphocytes. *Immunol. Rev.*, 111–156.
128. Malek, T. R., Clark, R. B., and Shevach, E. M. (1981): Alloreactive T cells from individual soft agar colonies specific for Guinea pig Ia antigens. I Production and initial characterization. *J. Immunol.*, 127:616–621.
129. Metcalf, D., Warner, N. L., Nossal, G. J. V., Miller, J. F. A. P., Shortman, D., and Rabellino, E. E. (1975): Growth of B-lymphocyte colonies in vitro from mouse lymphoid organs. *Nature*, 255:630–632.
130. Metcalf, D., Wilson, J. W., Shortman, K., Miller, J. F. A. P., and Stocker, J. (1978): The nature of the cells generating B-lymphocyte colonies in vitro. *J. Cell Physiol.*, 88:107–116.
131. Lala, P. K., and Johnson, G. R. (1978): Monoclonal origin of B lymphocyte colony-forming cells in spleen colonies formed by multipotential hemopoietic stem cells. *J. Exp. Med.*, 148:1468–1477.
132. Scott, D. W., Layton, J. E., and Johnson, G. R. (1978): Surface immunoglobulin phenotype of murine spleen cells which form B cell colonies in agar. *Eur. J. Immunol.*, 8:286–288.
133. Metcalf, D. (1976): Role of mercaptoethanol and endotoxin in stimulating B lymphocyte colony formation in vitro, *J. Immunol.*, 116:635–638.
134. Ulmer, A., and Maaurer, H. R. (1978): The formation of B-lymphocyte colonies in agar contained in glass capillaries. *Immunology*, 10:919–926.
135. Rozenszajn, L. A., Michlin, H., Kalechman, Y., and Sredni, B. (1977): Colony growth in vitro of mitogen-stimulated mouse B lymphocytes. *J. Immunol.*, 32:319.
136. Kincade, P. W., Ralph, P., and Moore, M. A. S. (1977): Regulation of B-lymphocyte clonal proliferation by stimulatory and inhibitory macrophage-derived factors. *J. Exp. Med.*, 146:1420–1435.
137. Kincade, P. W., Paige, C. J., Parkhouse, M. E., and Lee, G. (1978): Characterization of murine colony-forming B cells I. Distribution, resistance to anti-immunoglobulin antibodies and expression of Ia antigens. *J. Immunol.*, 120:947–953.
138. Kurland, J. I. (1978): Regulatory interactions of the macrophage in B-lymphocyte proliferation. *J. R. E. S.*, 24:19–26.
139. Jennings, G., and Shortman, K. (1982): Antigen-initiated B lymphocyte differentiation. XX. Colony-forming B lymphocytes are not identical with intermediate, "preprogenitor" subtest of primary or secondary B cells. *J. Immunol.*, 128:2095–2100.
140. Robak, D., and Whisler, R. (1980): Human B lymphocyte colony responses. I. General characteristics and modulation by monocytes. *J. Immunol.*, 125:2764–2769.
141. Whisler, R. L., Bobak, D. A., and Newhouse, V. G. (1981): Human B lymphocyte colony responses. II. The role of T cells in the enhancement of colony growth. *J. Immunol.*, 127:1758–1762.
142. Srendi, B., Sieckmann, D. G., Kumagai, S., House, S., Green, I., and Paul, W. I. (1981): Longterm culture and cloning of nortransformed human B lymphocytes. *J. Exp. Med.*, 154:1500–1516.
143. Lindahl-Kiessling, K., and Karlberg, I. (1982): Unicellular or multicellular origin of human T-lymphocyte colonies in soft agar? *Scand. J. Immunol.*, 15:525–530.
144. Farcet, J. P., and Testa, V. (1982): Human primary lymphocyte colony formation in agar culture. Polyclonal origin and significance. *Exp. Hematol.*, 10:172–177.
145. Singer, J. W., Ernst, C., Whaler, C. K., Steinmann, L., and Fiaikow, P. J. (1981): Single or multicellular origin of human T-lymphocyte colonies in-vitro. Modification by 12-0-tetradecanoyl phorbol 13 acetate. *J. Immunol.*, 126:1390–1392.
146. Klein, B., Caraux, J., Causse, A., Thierry, C., and Serrov, B. (1981): Human T-lymphocyte colonies. I. Surface markers and cytotoxic potential of colonies. *Biomedicine*, 34:34–39.
147. Ching, L-M., and Miller, R. G. (1981): Generation of cytotoxic T-lymphocyte precursor cells in T cell colonies in vitro. *Nature*, 289:802–804.
148. Klein, B., Caraux, J., Thierry, C., Gauci, L., Causse, A., and Serrov. B. (1981): Human T-lymphocyte colonies: Generation of colonies in different lymphocyte subpopulations. *Immunology*, 43:39–46.
149. Claesson, M. H., Sunderstrop-Hansen, G., and Poulsen, P. B. (1981): Colony formation by subpopulations of human T-lymphocytes. 2. Characteristics of colony cells and colony suppressor cells. *Scand. J. Immunol.*, 13:395–400.
150. Rozenszajn, L. A., Zeevi, A., Gopes, J., Radnay, J., and Sredni, B. (1978): Lymphocyte colony growth in vitro. *In: Hematopoietic Cell Differentiation* edited by D. W. Golde, M. J. Cline, D. Metcalf, and D. F. Fox, pp. 261–275. Academic Press, New York.

151. Srendi, B., Michlin, H., Kalechman, V., and Rozenszajn, L. A. (1978): Regulatory effects of macrophage secreted factors on thymus derived lymphocyte colony growth. *Cell Immunol.*, 36:15–27.
152. Krajewski, A. S., and Wyllie, A. H. (1981): Inhibition of human T-lymphocyte colony formation by methyl prednisolone. *Clin. Exp. Immunol.*, 46:206–213.
153. Eckels, D. D., and Gershwin, M. E. (1981): Pharmacologic and biochemical modulation of human T-lymphocyte colony formation. Hormonal influences. *Immunopharmacology*, 3:259–274.
154. Scharre, K. A., Eckels, D. D., and Gershwin, M. E. (1981): Depression of colony formation by human T-lymphocytes with rifampin and other antimicrobial agents. *J. Infect. Dis.*, 143:832–835.
155. Foa, R., and Catovsky, D. (1981): Inhibitory effect of cyclosporin A on peripheral blood and bone marrow T-lymphocyte colony formation. *Clin. Exp. Immunol.*, 45:371–375.
156. Gordon, M. Y. (1981): Effect of levamisole on T-lymphocyte colony formation by cells from bone marrow aspirates. *Clin. Exp. Immunol.*, 45:365–370.
157. Herrod, H. G., and Valenski, W. R. (1981): T-lymphocyte colony forming capacity of patients with immunodeficiency diseases: Relationship of colony formation to erythrocyte rosette formation and lymphocyte proliferation. *Clin. Exp. Immunol.*, 45:562–567.
158. Eckels, D. D., and Gershwin, M. E. (1981): T-lymphocyte colony formation and autoimmune disease. In vitro assessment of immunopathology. *J. Rheumatol.*, 8:214–219.
159. Kurland, J. I., Kincade, P. W., and Moore, M. A. S. (1977): Regulation of bone marrow derived lymphocyte clonal proliferation by stimulatory and inhibitory macrophage derived factors. *J. Exp. Med.*, 146:1420–1435.
160. Hara, H., and Ogawa, M. (1978): Murine hemopoietic colonies in culture containing normoblasts, macrophages and megakaryocytes. *Am. J. Hematol.*, 4:23–27.
161. Fauser, A. A., and Messner, H. A. (1978): Granulocrythropoietic colonies in human bone marrow, peripheral blood and cord blood. *Blood*, 52:1243–1248.
162. Fauser, A. A., and Messner, H. A. (1979): Identification of megakaryocytes, macrophages, and eosinophils in colonies of human bone marrow containing neutrophilic granulocytes and erthroblasts. *Blood*, 53:1023–1030.
163. Messner, H. A., Izaquirre, C. A., and Jamal, N. (1982): Identification of T-lymphocytes in human mixed hemopoietic colonies *Blood*, 58:402–405.
164. Metcalf, D., and Johnson, G. R. (1978): Mixed hemopoietic colonies in vitro. *In: Hematopoietic Cell Differentiation*, edited by D. W. Golde, D. Metcalf, and C. F. Fox, pp. 141–151. Academic Press, New York.
165. Messner, H. A., Izaquirre, C. A., and Jamal, N. (1981): Identification of T-lymphocytes in human mixed hemopoietic colonies. *Blood*, 58:402–405.
166. Hara, H. (1983): Presence of cells in B-cell lineage in mixed (GEMM) colonies from murine marrow cells. *Int. J. Cell Cloning*, 1:171–178.
167. Ogawa, M., and Porter, P. N. (1983): Gross hierarchy of hemopoietic stem cells assayable in culture: Statistical analysis of their self-renewal and differentiation. *J. Cell. Biochem.*, *[Suppl.]* 713:8.
168. Nakahata, T., and Ogawa, M. J. (1982): Clonal origin of murine hemopoietic colonies with apparent restriction to granulocyte-macrophage-megakaryocyte (GMM) differentiation. *J. Cell. Physiol.*, 111:239–245.
169. Dexter, T. M., Allen, T. D., Lajtha, L. G., Schofield, R., and Lord, B. I. (1973): Stimulation of differentiation and proliferation of haemopoietic cells in vitro. *J. Cell. Physiol.*, 82:461–473.
170. Dexter, T. M., Spooncer, E., Hendry, J., and Lajtha, L. G. (1978): Stem cells in vitro. *In: Hematopoietic Cell Differentiation*. edited by D. W. Golde, M. J. Cline, D. Metcalf, and C. F. Fox, pp. 163–173, Academic Press, New York.
171. Testa, N. G., and Dexter, T. M. (1978): Long-term production of erythroid cells (BFU) in bone marrow cultures. *Differentiation*, 9:193–195.
172. Williams, N., Jackson, H., Sheridan, A. P. C., Murphy, M. J., Jr., Elste, A., and Moore, M. A. S. (1978): Regulation of megakaryopoiesis in long-term murine bone marrow cultures. *Blood*, 51:245–255.
173. Dexter, T. M., Moore, M. A. S., and Sheridan, A. P. C. (1977): Maintenance of hemopoietic stem cells and production of differentiated progeny in allogeneic and semi-allogeneic bone marrow chimeras in vitro. *J. Exp. Med.*,145:1612–1616.
174. Eastmen, C. E., and Ruscetti, F. W. (1982): Evaluation of erythropoiesis in long-term hamster bone marrow suspension cultures. *Blood*, 60:999–1006.

175. Weiss, L. (1976): The hematopoietic microenvironment of the bone marrow: An ultrastructural study of the stroma in rats. *Anat. Rec.*, 196:161–184.

176. Greenberger, J. (1978): Sensitivity of corticosteroid-dependent insulin-resistant lipogenesis in marrow preadipocytes of obese-diabetic (db/db) mice. *Nature*, 275:752–754.

177. Westen, H., and Bainton, D. F. (1979): Association of alkaline-phosphatase-positive reticulum cells in bone marrow with granulocytic precursors. *J. Exp. Med.*, 150:919–937.

178. Greenberg, B. R., Wilson, F. D., Woo, L., and Jenks, H. M. (1978): Cytogenetics of fibroblastic colonies in Ph¹-positive chronic myelogenous leukemia. *Blood*, 51:1039–1044.

179. Patt, H. M., and Maloney, M. A. (1975): Bone marrow regeneration after local injury: A review. *Exp. Hematol.*, 3:135–148.

180. Patt, H. M., Maloney, M. A., and Flannery, M. L. (1982): Hematopoietic microenvironment transfer by stromal fibroblasts derived from bone marrow varying in cellularity. *Exp. Hematol.*, 10:738–742.

181. Bernstein, S. E. (1970): Tissue transplantation as an analytic and theraputic tool in hereditery anemias. *Am. J. Surg.*, 119:448.

182. Knospe, W. H., Blom, J., and Crosby, W. H. (1966): Regeneration of locally irradiated bone marrow. I. Dose dependent, long-term changes in the rat with particular emphasis upon vascular and stromal reaction. *Blood*, 28:398–415.

183. McCulloch, E. A., Siminovitch, L., Till, J. E., Russel, E. A., and Bernstein, S. E. (1965): The cellulor basis of the genetically determined hemopoietic defect in anemic mice of genotype sl/sl^d. *Blood*, 26:399–410.

184. Wolf, N. S. (1974): Dissecting the hematopoietic micro-environment. I. Stem cell lodgement and commitment, and proliferation and differentiation of erythropoietic descendents in the sl/sl^d mouse. *Cell Tissue Kinet.*, 7:89–94.

185. Wilson, F. D., Stitzel, K. A., Klein, A. K., Shifrine, M., Graham, R., Jones, M., Bradley, E. W., and Rosenblatt, L. S. (1978): Quantitative response of bone marrow colony-forming units (CFU-C and PFU-C) in weaning beagles exposed to acute whole-body gamma-irradiation. *Radiat. Res.*, 74:289–297.

186. Tavassoli, M., and Crosby, W. H. (1968): Transplantation of marrow to extramedullary sites. *Science*, 161:54–55.

187. Friedenstein, A. J., Petrakooa, K. V., Kurolesqua, A. I., and Frolova, G. E. (1968): Heterotopic transplants of bone marrow. *Transplantation*, 6:230–247.

188. Wilson, F. D., Greenberg, B. R., Konrad, P. N., Klein, A. K., and Walling, P. A. (1978): Cytogenetic studies on bone marrow fibroblasts from a male-female hematopoietic chimera. *Transplantation*, 25:87–88.

189. Golde, D., Hocking, W. G., Quan, S. G., Sparkes, R. S., and Gala, R. P. (1980): Origin of human bone marrow fibroblasts. *Br. J. Haematol.*, 44:183–187.

190. Bentley, S. A., and Foident, J-M. (1980): Some properties of marrow derived adherent cells in tissue culture. *Blood*, 56:1006–1012.

191. Friedenstein, A. J., Ivanor-Smolenski, A. A., Chajlakjan, R. K., Gorskaya, V. R., Kuralesova, A. I., and Latzinik, N. W. (1978): Gera simon, U.N. Origin of bone marrow stromal mechanocytes in radiochimeras and heterotopic transplants. *Exp. Hematol.*, 6:440–444.

192. Maximow, A. A. (1926-27): Development of nogranulor leukocytes (lymphocytes and monocytes) into polyblasts (macrophages) and fibroblasts in vitro. *Proc. Soc. Exp. Biol. Med.*, 24:570–572.

193. Wilson, F. D., Tavassoli, M., Greenberg, D., Hinds, D., and Klein, A. K. (1981): Morphological studies in adherent cells in bone marrow cultures from humans, dogs and mice. *Stem Cells*, 1:15–19.

194. Castro-Malaspina, H., Gay, R. E., Resnick, G., Kapoor, N., Meyers, P., Chiarieri, D., McKenzie, S., Broxmeyer, H. E., and Moore, M. A. S. (1980): Characterization of human bone marrow fibroblast colony-forming cells (CFU-F) and their progeny. *Blood*, 56:289–301.

195. Greenberg, B. R., Wilson, F. D., and Woo, L. (1981): Granulopoietic effects of human bone marrow fibroblastic cells and abnormalities in the granulopoietic microenvironment. *Blood*, 58:557–564.

196. Wilson, F. D., and O'Grady, L. (1976): Some observations on the hematopoietic status in vivo and in vitro in mice of genotype S1/S1^d. *Blood*, 48:601–608.

197. Wilson, F. D., Greenberg, B. R., Spangler, W., Shifrine, M., Gershwin, M. E., and Dyck, J. (1978): Production of mesenchymal tumors in nude mice by Ph¹-negative fibroblasts obtained from a Ph¹-positive CML patient. *Exp. Hematol.*, 6:549–557.

198. Wilson, F. D., Greenberg, B. R., Spangler, W. L., Shifrine, M., and Gershwin, M. E. (1978): Production of mesenchymal tumors in nude mice using Ph¹ negative "fibroblasts" obtained from a Ph¹ positive CML patient and other human sources. *In: Hematopoietic Cellular Differentiation*, edited by D. W. Golde, M. J. Cline, and D. Metcalf, pp. 231–240, Academic Press, New York.

199. Wilson, F. D., Gershwin, M. E., Shifrine, M., and Graham, R. (1977): Increased clonogenic (CFU-C, PFU-C) populations from bone marrow and spleen of nude mice. *Dev. Comp. Immunol.*, 1:373–384.

200. Werts, E. D., DeGowin, R. L., Knapp, S. K., and Gibson, D. P. (1980): Characterization of marrow stomal (fibroblastoid) cells and their association with erythropoiesis. *Exp. Hemat.*, 8:423–433.

201. Greenberg, B. R., Wilson, F. D., Woo, L., Klein, A. K., and Rosenblatt, L. S. (1984): Increased in vitro radioresistance of bone marrow fibroblastic cells from patients with acute nonlymphocytic leukemia. *Leukemia Res. (in press.)*

202. Bauldry, S. A., Wilson, F. D., and Ackerman, G. A. (1983): The stimulation of rat bone marrow fibroblast colony formation by 2 merceptoethanol. *Int. J. Cell Colony*, 1:151–158.

203. Greenberg, B. R., Wilson, F. D., and Woo, L. (1981): Cytogenetic analysis and granulopoietic effects of bone marrow fibroblastic colonies in Fanconi's anemia. *Br. J. Haematol.*, 48:85.

204. Bauldry, S. A., Wilson, F. D., Stromberg, P. C., Ackerman, G. A. (1983): The effects of Fisher rat leukemic serum on bone marrow fibroblast colony formation. *J. Cell. Biochem., [Suppl.]* 78:41.

205. Groopman, J. E. (1980): The pathogenesis of myelofibrosis in myeloproliferative disorders. *Ann. Int. Med.*, 92:857–859.

206. Castro-Malaspina, H., Rabellino, E. M., Yen, A., Nachman, R. L., and Moore, M. A. S. (1981): Human megakaryocyte stimulation of proliferation of bone marrow fibroblasts. *Blood*, 57:781–787.

207. Ershler, W. B., Ross, J., Finlay, J. L., and Shanhidi, N. T. (1980): Bone marrow microenvironment defect on congenital hypoplastic anemia. *N. Engl. J. Med.*, 302:1321–1326.

208. Gordon, M. Y., and Gordon-Smith (1981): Bone marrow fibroblastoid colony-forming cells (F-CFC) in aplastic anemia: Colony growth and stimulation of granulocyte-macrophage colony-forming cells (GM-CFC) *Br. J. Haematol.*, 49:465–477.

209. Wiktor-Jedrzejcak, W., Slekierzynski, M., Szcaylik, C., Gornas, P., and Dryjanski, T. (1982): Aplastic anemia with marrow defective in formation of fibroblastoid cell colonies in vitro. *Scand. J. Haematol.*, 28:82–90.

210. DeGowin, R. L., and Gibson, D. P. (1978): Suppressive effects of an extramedullory tumor on bone marrow erythropoiesis and stroma. *Exp. Hematol.*, 6:568–575.

211. Werts, E. D., Gibson, D. P., and DeGowin, R. L. (1979): Chronic inflammation suppresses bone marrow stromal cells and medullury erythropoiesis. *J. Clin. Med.*, 93:995–1001.

212. Castro-Malaspina, H., Gay, R. E., Jhanwor, S. C., Hamilton, J. A., Chiareri, D., Meyers, P. A., Gay, S., and Moore, M. A. S. (1982): Characteristics of bone marrow fibroblast colony-forming cell (CFU-C) and their progeny in patients with myeloproliferative disorders. *Blood*, 59:1046–1053.

213. Ben-Ishay, Z., Bornstein, A., Sharon, S., and Prindull, G. (1983): Incidence and characteristics of colony-forming unit fibroblasts (CFU-C) in the bone marrow of weanling mice treated with cytosine arabinoside and phenylhydrazine; correlation with CFU-S, progenitors of diffusion-chamber colonies (CFU-D) and CFU-C. *Int. J. Cell. Cloning*, 1:343–348.

Toxicology of the Blood and Bone Marrow,
edited by Richard D. Irons. Raven Press,
New York © 1985.

Flow Cytofluorometric Analysis of Blood and Bone Marrow

Richard D. Irons and Wayne S. Stillman

Chemical Industry Institute of Toxicology, Research Triangle Park, North Carolina 27709

Normal hemopoiesis is characterized by an ordered process of proliferation and differentiation in bone marrow precursor cell populations, beginning with the pluripotent stem cell and terminating in the production of mature end-stage blood cells. Evolution of our knowledge of the structure and function of the bone marrow in hemopoiesis has been accompanied by an increasingly sophisticated array of methods and approaches, many of which have been discussed in previous chapters. Examples of these are the *in vivo* and *in vitro* stem cell assays and the kinetic methods previously described to study bone marrow precursor and transit cell populations. A rapidly expanding technology that offers additional potential to study function, growth, and differentiation in hemopoietic cells is flow cytofluorometry. The application of this instrumental technique, together with the contribution of monoclonal antibody technology, has tremendously influenced hematology and immunology research and has the potential to greatly accelerate toxicologic investigation in these areas as well.

Flow cytofluorometry (FCF) permits the quantitative measurement of a variety of properties on individual cells in a flow stream at rates of several thousand cells per second. FCF, flow cytometer, flow microfluorometer (FMF), fluorescence-activated cell sorter (FACS), laser-based multiparameter cell sorter, and electronically programmable individual cell sorter (EPICS) are all terms used variously to describe similar types of instrumentation. Examples of parameters that can be measured on individual cells include single or dual wavelength fluorescence, low-angle and 90 degree-angle light scatter, cell number, and cell volume. A major advantage of this technique is that in addition to making stochastic measurements on populations of cells, it permits the study of multiparameter data that is individually correlated for single cells. Since more than one parameter can be measured on individual cells at rates, in some cases as high as 5,000/sec, cell population distributions can be studied with a high degree of statistical significance.

INSTRUMENTATION AND SAMPLE PREPARATION

The basic design of the FCF is similar in principle to that of a fluorometer, the major components being an excitation source, a means of sample containment, and a detector(s) (Fig. 1). Measurements on individual cells are made by introducing a suspension of cells via a laminar flow chamber such that the cells pass through in single file. A source of high-energy excitation is required, usually either a tunable laser or a mercury arc lamp. In a majority of instruments cells in a flow stream are passed through a laser beam and detection of fluorescence or scattered light accomplished using photoelectric detectors placed perpendicular to the exciting light beam. In laser-based instruments specificity of excitation is obtained by using monochromatic light of a particular wavelength and appropriate barrier filter combinations. Single and dual laser instruments are commercially available, the latter enabling simultaneous excitation at two different wavelengths for multiple-parameter fluorescence analysis. An additional feature of the cell sorter is its ability to sort individual cells on the basis of their fluorescence or light scatter distribution patterns. In sorting instruments the flow stream is vibrated at a given frequency to induce the uniform formation of droplets containing single cells. Droplets containing cells that satisfy predetermined sort criteria are charged and deflected by an electrostatic field into an appropriate collection device. This brief description is intended to provide an introduction to the basic instrument. Expansion of hardware in this field over the last few years has been logarithmic, and a comprehensive description of various instrument configurations and features commercially available is beyond the scope of this chapter. Shapiro recently published an excellent history of the development of commercial instrumentation in flow cytometry and its implications for research in biology (45).

Suspensions of individual cells are required for FCF analysis or sorting. Cells may be suspended in any aqueous solution (buffer, media, etc.). Blood, bone marrow, and lymphoid cells are readily dispersed by mechanical aspiration whereas other tissues may require more strenuous methods. Tissue or culture samples can be freshly suspended and analyzed directly or subjected to fractionation procedures to obtain standardized or enriched populations of selected cells (23,40).

PARAMETERS

Light Scatter Measurements

When a cell or particle passes through a beam of coherent light such as a laser beam, measurement of the light scattered in the forward direction (0.5° to 20°) or at right angles (90°) to the beam can be a useful parameter for the discrimination of hematopoietic cell populations. Light scattered in the forward direction is due, in large part, to diffraction from surfaces or biologic membranes. Forward angle light scatter is theoretically proportional to the diameter of the cell, and with certain reservations can be used to discriminate cell populations on the basis of size. Low angle light scatter is also influenced by the refractive index of a cell, and the measurement is often used to discriminate between live and dead cells. This is important for immunofluorescence analysis because of the characteristic increase in nonspecific binding of immunoglobulin associated with dead cells that

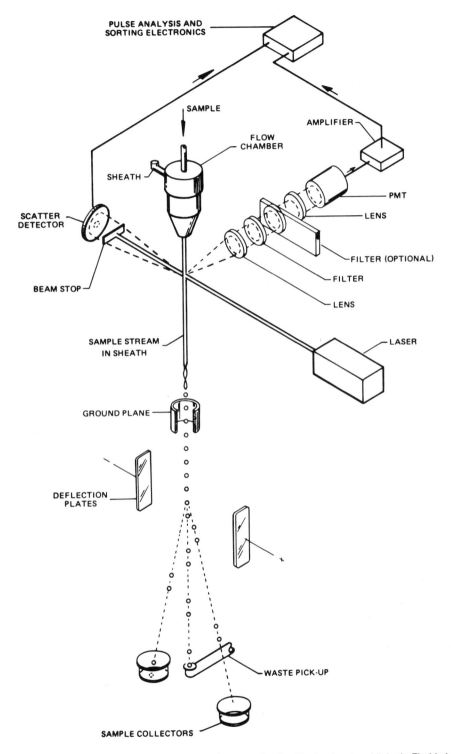

FIG. 1. Basic components of a cell sorter. (Courtesy Coulter Electronics, Inc., Hialeah, Florida.)

can contribute to or interfere with specific immunofluorescence measurements. It should be pointed out, however, that light scatter as a monitor of cell death may be less sensitive than dye exclusion methods (9,41) and requires a relatively homogeneous cell population with respect to size. Similar to its use as an indicator of cell size, the utility of low angle light scatter as an indicator of cell viability must be evaluated for use in each application. Right angle or orthogonal light scatter measurements are, to a large extent, dependent on internal cell structures. The simultaneous determination of orthogonal and forward angle light scatter is of use in discriminating different bone marrow and blood cell populations (Fig. 2).

Fluorescence Measurements

The majority of FCF methods to date are based on fluorescence measurements and are predicated either on the measurement of intrinsic fluorescent molecules or on the uptake and/or binding of a fluorescent substance to specific structures on or in the cell. Fluorescence intensity emitted from an excited cell will be the summation of the intrinsic fluorescence of the cell and the emission intensity of a molecular probe for any given excitation wavelength. Virtually any intracellular substance or surface membrane structure for which an appropriate fluorescent probe exists can be quantitated. The two most frequent applications to date have been the analysis of individual cell DNA content using fluorescent probes and the determination of cell surface antigenic properties by immunofluorescence. Other substances that have been quantitated in individual cells include protein (17,24), RNA (49,50), and individual enzyme activities using substrates that yield fluorescent products (14,39).

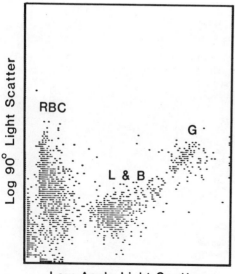

FIG. 2. Two-dimensional scattergram of 90° versus low angle light scatter for freshly isolated murine bone marrow cells. Isolated population distributions correspond to (RBC) erythrocytes; (L&B) lymphoid and blast cells; (G) granulocyte and macrophages.

DNA Cell Cycle Analysis

Cell cycle analysis by FCF is based on the ability to quantitate DNA content in individual cells. Cell suspensions are stained with fluorescent compounds that stoichiometrically bind to DNA and therefore yield staining intensities proportional to the individual cell's DNA content. Examples of dyes that have been used for this purpose include the interchelating dyes, ethidium bromide and propidium iodide, the so-called "groove binding" antibiotics mithramycin and chromomycin, the Hoechst-Roussel dyes and 4',6-diamidino-2-phenylindole (DAPI). Latt provides an exceptionally complete review of these compounds and their application (33). The normal life cycle of the cell can be divided into four discrete phases on the basis of DNA synthesis: M, mitosis; G_0/G_1, the first gap or period of no measurable DNA synthesis; S, the phase of measurable DNA synthesis; and, G_2, the second period of no measurable DNA synthesis (Fig. 3).

Normal bone marrow precursor cells are characterized as undergoing asynchronous exponential growth. Cells move through the cycle independent of one another, and the transit time for any given phase of the cycle is independent of the transit time for any other. In any given cohort of bone marrow cells the probability that a cycling cell will be in a particular phase of the cell cycle is then proportional to the amount of the total cell cycle transit time spent in that phase. The theoretical distribution histogram for DNA content in an asynchronous exponentially growing cell population is shown in Fig. 4A. The phases of no DNA synthesis are represented by single values for individual cell DNA content, G_2 phase cells containing exactly twice the amount of DNA as G_1/G_0 cells. Cells in mitosis contain exactly the same amount of DNA as G_2 cells and are therefore indistinguishable on the

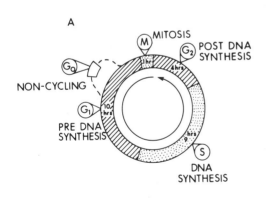

FIG. 3. Representation of DNA cell cycle based on hypothetical 24-hr transit time. (Reprinted from Irons, ref. 25, with permission.)

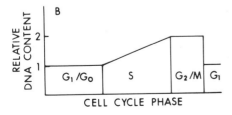

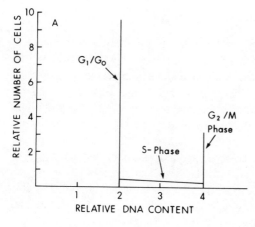

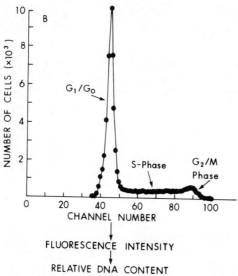

FIG. 4. DNA distribution. **A:** Theoretical histogram for population of cells in asynchronous exponential growth. **B:** Actual histogram obtained by cytofluorometric analysis of freshly isolated rabbit bone marrow cells stained with mithramycin. (Modified from Irons, ref. 25, with permission.)

basis of DNA content. Cells in S phase are represented by a linear continuum of values for DNA content. An experimentally determined histogram of cells isolated from normal rabbit bone marrow illustrates the experimental error contributed by biologic variability among different cell types, instrumental stability, and lack of proportionality between DNA content and fluorescence intensity (Fig. 4B).

Although simple arithmetic methods exist for obtaining estimates of the proportion of cycling cells in a given population, most laboratories employ some form of computer-based mathematical analysis to determine the proportion of cells in various phases of the cell cycle. These include parametric as well as nonparametric methods that have been well described elsewhere (1,13,18,46). The selection of one method over another depends on a number of factors and should be influenced by the various experimental assumptions on which each method is based. In practice the choice is usually made empirically, depending on the precision with which the various methods approximate the raw histogram data.

CELL SURFACE MARKER ANALYSIS

Analysis of cell surface antigens by FCF has become an important technique for identifying bone marrow and lymphoid cell populations and studying cell differentiation. Immunofluorescence labeling of cell surface antigens is accomplished by directly or indirectly binding a fluorescent probe to an antibody with specificity toward the cell surface determinants of interest. The most well-known and time-honored method involves the direct conjugation of antibody with fluorescein using fluorescein isothiocyanate (FITC) or rhodamine (45). Antibody-sandwich labeling methods refer to the use of a second fluorescent-labeled antibody directed against the first antibody which is bound to the cell surface antigen. Sandwich or indirect labeling methods can be highly advantageous and are usually a necessity when simultaneous labeling of multiple surface antigens is desired. However, a practical limitation of the use of anti-antibody secondary reagents stems from the fact that most monoclonals directed against cell surface antigens are derived from mouse or rat hybridomas and are mouse or rat immunoglobulin, usually IgG. Therefore, the use of secondary antibodies is restricted by the limited variety of immunoglobulins represented by primary reagents. Adding to the problem is the fact that antibodies directed toward either mouse or rat Ig often exhibit at least some minimal cross-reactivity with each other or human Ig. Fortunately, additional indirect labeling techniques are available that do not involve secondary anti-antibody reagents. These include avidin-biotin and arsenilate-anti-arsenilate labeling methods as well as a wide range of other hapten-based sandwich techniques (55).

APPLICATIONS

Bone Marrow Cell Cycle Kinetics

Cells may demonstrate sensitivity to cytotoxic agents depending on their position in the cell cycle. Cycle-specific agents may act directly on cells in a particular phase of the cycle, although the phase of maximum sensitivity may or may not correspond to the phase of arrest or cell death (37). It was established by E. Beutler *(this volume)* that cycle-specific agents such as methotrexate produce a dose-survival curve with a plateau above which no increase in cytotoxicity is observed with increasing dose. This occurs because exposure to such agents results in a partial synchronization of the target cell population. Surviving cells are spared because of their position in the cell cycle, the proportion of which will remain constant for a given exposure regimen.

Cytofluorometric analysis of DNA provides an exceedingly sensitive method for determining the effects of chemical exposure on cell cycle kinetics. We have previously used this technique to determine the effects of benzene on dividing bone marrow cells. Like colchicine, benzene is an example of an agent that appears to induce cycle-specific changes in proliferating bone marrow cell populations (Fig. 5). Both of these compounds are mitotic spindle poisons, blocking cells in G_2/M of the cell cycle; however, sensitivity to the cytotoxic effects of these agents appears to be restricted to cells undergoing microtubule synthesis during S phase (25,26,38).

Cell Activation and Blastogenesis

An interesting application with potential utility in studying the effects of chemical exposure on early events in blastogenesis involves the measurement of intrinsic substances that are correlated with these events. Examples include the simultaneous quantitation of RNA and DNA; quantitative analysis of surface antigens, such as transferrin receptors, whose appearance is associated with the deterministic commitment to cell division in G_1; and the measurement of early events in cell activation that immediately follow receptor-ligand interaction at the cell surface, such as the

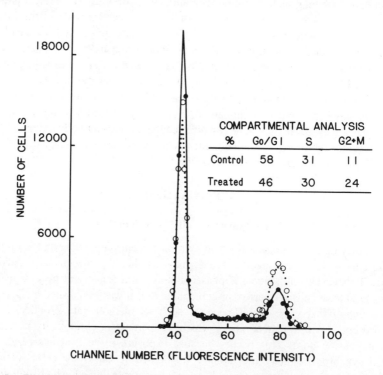

FIG. 5. Effects of benzene treatment on DNA cell cycle phase in rabbit bone marrow. Representative DNA distribution for a control rabbit injected subcutaneously once a day with corn oil *(closed circles)* or with 0.3 ml/kg/day benzene in corn oil *(open circles)* for 3 days. Bone marrow aspirates were obtained 24 hr after the last injection; cells purified by density gradient centrifugation and stained with mithramycin. Compartmental analysis was performed using a modification of the Fried algorithm (18).

flux of Ca^{2+} across the plasma membrane and alterations in plasma membrane potential.

Acridine orange has been employed for the simultaneous measurement of RNA and DNA because its emission profile is different, depending on whether it is bound to single- or double-stranded nucleic acid. Using this technique Darzynkiewicz and co-workers demonstrated that cells in G_0/G_1 can be subdivided into distinct subpopulations on the basis of their RNA content, which, in turn, correlates with their level of activation or commitment to enter S phase (6,10,11). A two-parameter DNA/RNA distribution scattergram obtained by staining freshly isolated murine spleen cells with acridine orange is presented in Fig. 6. Cellular RNA content is known to increase during S phase such that G_2/M cells contain twice the complement of RNA of G_1 cells. However, G_1 cells can be divided into two compartments on the basis of RNA content, those that contain the minimum RNA content of S phase cells and those that contain approximately 20% less RNA. A number of experiments suggest that G_1 cells containing the minimum RNA content of S-phase cells represent cells committed to entry into S phase (10). This technique may facilitate studies of the early events in a cell's commitment to blastogenesis and can be used to study the effects of various agents on the early stages of cell proliferation.

Expression of transferrin receptors on the cell surface is closely linked with proliferation in both normal and neoplastic cells (29,31,32). Furthermore, a lymphoma-transforming gene has been shown to code for a protein-sharing homology with transferrin (19). Transferrin receptor expression is therefore a potentially useful indicator of cell activation. Figure 7 illustrates the appearance of transferrin receptors on murine splenic lymphocytes following mitogen stimulation in culture with phytohemagglutinin.

Studies by Shapiro and others suggest that cytofluorometric analysis of membrane potential and Ca^{2+} flux may prove useful in studying the effects of physical or chemical agents in altering the growth and differentiation of cell populations in culture (44). These techniques are based on the use of fluorescent chelators of

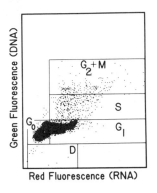

FIG. 6. Two-parameter DNA/RNA scattergram for freshly isolated murine spleen cells. Cells were stained with acridine orange, excited at a wavelength of 488 nm, and analyzed simultaneously for DNA (green fluorescence, 530 nm) and RNA (red fluorescence, 640) by FCF. D, dead cells.

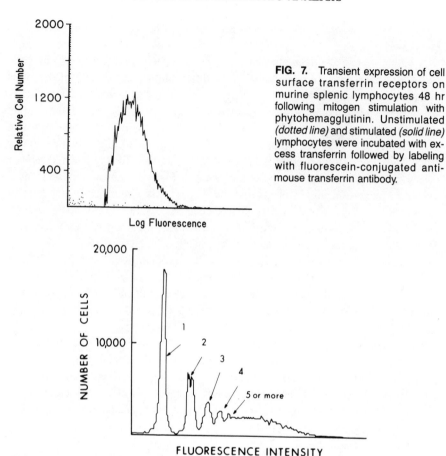

FIG. 7. Transient expression of cell surface transferrin receptors on murine splenic lymphocytes 48 hr following mitogen stimulation with phytohemagglutinin. Unstimulated *(dotted line)* and stimulated *(solid line)* lymphocytes were incubated with excess transferrin followed by labeling with fluorescein-conjugated anti-mouse transferrin antibody.

FIG. 8. Phagocytosis of fluorescein-labeled latex beads by murine splenic macrophages *in vitro*. Phagocytized fluorescent microspheres (2.0 μ). (Modified from Irons et al., ref. 27, with permission.)

Ca^{2+}, such as chlorotetracycline and a variety of lipophilic cationic dyes that partition across the plasma membrane as a function of membrane potential.

Lymphoid and Hemopoietic Cell Function

A variety of methods are available for assessing terminal differentiation or end-stage cell function, examples of which include: phagocytosis, antibody production, cell-mediated cytotoxicity or cytostasis, macrophage activation, and chemoluminescence. Most have been developed for the analysis of lymphoid and macrophage populations. Phagocytosis is quantitated by monitoring the quantal increase in fluorescence accompanying the phagocytosis of uniform fluorescent latex particles (27,35,48). Figure 8 illustrates the ability of the technique to enumerate macrophages on the basis of the quantitative assessment of phagocytized fluorescent microspheres. A potential difficulty with this method relates to distinguishing between phagocytized and surface-bound particles; the latter apparently are not uniformly removed by subjecting the cells to enzymatic digestion or calcium chelation procedures (R. Parod, *personal communication*). Target-cell killing by activated lymphoid or macrophage populations can be monitored by measuring cytostasis (DNA cell cycle analysis) if the target cell population is normally in asynchronous exponential growth (see ref. 27) or by determining viability (D. E. Lewis, *personal communication*). Cell viability can be measured using dye exclusion (7,22) or vital staining (41) techniques. In the former, uptake of a molecule normally impermeable to intact membranes is used as an indicator of membrane degeneration and thus cell death. Examples of probes useful for this purpose are the DNA stains, ethidium bromide, mithramycin, and propidium iodide. Vital staining, which in our hands appears to be more sensitive than dye exclusion methods, can be achieved by using compounds such as fluorescein diacetate, which is readily taken up by living cells; upon enzymatic liberation, the fluorescein molecule becomes impermeable and trapped within the cell. The loss of fluorescence with time, therefore, can be as a monitor of increased membrane permeability (41). Macrophage activation can be assessed by monitoring the altered density of selected surface antigen expression. Elicitation of activated macrophages by the phorbol ester, 12-0-tetra-decanoyl phorbol 13-acetate, is accompanied by changes in the density of the MAC-1 surface antigen on macrophages isolated from murine spleen (Fig. 9).

A number of instrumental techniques have been described and used for several years on prototype instruments and recently have become available on commercial instruments. These include time-of-flight, slit-scan optics, fluorescence polarization, and energy transfer. Time-of-flight, or pulse width analysis, refers to the electronic measurement of fluorescence signal pulse width, and, depending on variations in instrumental design, simultaneous determination of pulse height or pulse rise time (34). These measurements provide information on particle size and geometry. Slit-scan FCF refers to the use of narrow beam excitation to provide additional information on the distribution of fluorescence intensity across the

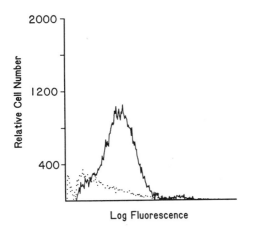

FIG. 9. Expression of MAC-1 surface marker on normal and activated murine splenic macrophages. Macrophages were obtained from mice injected intraperitoneally with corn oil *(dotted line)* or 20 μg/g 12-0-tetradecanoyl phorbol 13-acetate in corn oil twice a week for 2 weeks *(solid line)* and isolated by density gradient centrifugation.

diameter of a particle as it transmits the laser beam (54). Conventional FCF employs zero-resolution optics in which a particle is completely contained within the aperture of the exciting light source. With slit-scan FCF, the aperture of the exciting laser beam is either mechanically or optically reduced to a diameter less than that of the particle being measured (typically 1 to 4 μm). The measurement of fluorescence intensity versus time thus provides a contour profile of fluorescence distribution across the particle. Both of these techniques have been applied to the analysis of mammalian chromosomes (5,8,20). These techniques may prove useful for studying the dynamics of redistribution of cell surface receptors (patching, capping). Additional parameters include fluorescence polarization and energy transfer measurements, detailed discussion of which is beyond the scope of this chapter. These provide information on the orientation and proximity of molecules and can be used to probe the structure of cell membranes, membrane fluidity, and transmembrane control of molecules on the surface of the cell (28).

DNA Damage and Aneuploidy

A potentially interesting application of FCF DNA analysis to genetic toxicology studies is the analysis of aneuploidy and micronuclei in individual cells. Micronuclei are clumps of cytoplasmic nuclear chromatin that can occur as a result of the production of acentric chromosomal fragments or whole chromosomes lagging at anaphase. Aneuploidy refers to an abnormal number of chromosomes that are probably the result of nondisjunctional events occurring during anaphase. These abnormalities and their potential significance are discussed further in the chapter by R. R. Tice and J. L. Ivett *(this volume)*. Micronuclei, or Howell-Jolly bodies, are often manually enumerated in anucleated erythrocytes. FCF analysis of micronuclei in erythrocytes is based on the quantitative measurement of cytoplasmic DNA at concentrations less than that observed in normal diploid (G_1/G_0) cell nuclei. The relationship of sub-G_1/G_0 DNA cell content to cytologically identifiable cytoplasmic chromatin has not been rigorously validated; nevertheless, preliminary studies indicate FCF DNA analysis to be sufficiently sensitive to make such studies feasible. Hutter and Stohr, for example, have applied the simultaneous analysis of DNA and protein fluorochromes [4′-6′-diamidino′-2-phenylindole (DAPI) and sulforhodamine, respectively] to the determination of micronuclei in bone marrow (24). Alternatively, the simultaneous analysis of DNA and RNA using acridine orange or a combination of dyes, such as DAPI or Hoechst and the RNA stain, pyronin Y (49), should permit the cytofluorometric analysis of micronuclei in peripheral blood reticulocytes.

The analysis of aneuploidy in nucleated cell populations is of potentially major biologic importance since specific chromosomal deletions and rearrangements have been closely linked with a number of human malignancies. Theoretically, aneuploidy should alter the coefficient of variation about the G_1 peak; nevertheless, detection and analysis of multiple aneuploid G_1 peaks in DNA histograms require resolution of a considerably higher degree than is obtained using routine staining and curve stripping techniques. Schuette and co-workers recently described a feedback-controlled curve fitting procedure that permits the resolution of closely spaced multiple aneuploid G_1 peaks (43). Independently, Barlogie and co-workers (2,3) successfully measured aneuploidy in human leukemias and lymphomas using a specialized high-resolution pulse cytofluorometric technique.

Identification of Hemopoietic Cells and Analysis of Differentiation

The first subgrouping of lymphocytes into T and B cells using flow cytometry was performed by Kreth and Hertzenberg in 1974 (30). In the last 10 years numerous subpopulations of lymphoid and hemopoietic cells have been characterized by correlating cell surface antigens with cytology and/or cell function. Nothing approaching a complete array of reagents currently exists that would permit a thorough quantitation of hemopoietic cell lines on the basis of surface marker analysis; however, with the tremendous activity in this area the field is changing rapidly. Table 1 provides a partial listing of antibodies that are commercially available for the study of lymphoid and hemopoietic cells in man, mouse, and rat. It should be noted that several of these reagents, while reacting with antigenic determinants expressed on a particular cell population (e.g., bone marrow stem cells, macrophages, etc.), do not recognize these cell types exclusively. The reader should consult the literature on a specific reagent or antigen to determine appropriate use. A reasonably complete compendium of commercially available immunoreagents is *Linscott's Directory of Immunological and Biological Reagents* (36).

TABLE 1. *Partial list of commercially available monoclonal antibodies directed against lymphoid and hematopoietic cell lines*

Cell type	Human	Murine[a]	Rat
T cells (PAN-T)	Anti-Leu-1[b]; OKT11[c]	Anti-Thy	W3/13[d,e]
T helper/inducer	Anti-Leu-3; OKT4	Anti-Lyt-1	W3/25
T cytotoxic/suppressor	Anti-Leu-2; OKT8	Anti-Lyt2; Anti-Lyt3	OX8
B cells	Anti-Leu-12; OKB7	Anti-LyB1 - LyB7	
Natural killer cells	Anti-Leu-7; Anti-Leu-11		
Monocytes	Anti-Leu-M3; OKM1		
Macrophages	MAC-1(M1/70)[f]	MAC-1	
Granulocytes	Anti-Leu-M4; MAC-1	GM-1.2[g]; MAC-1	
Bone marrow stem cells	OKT10[e]		W3/13[e]

[a]All murine reagents listed designate antigenic determinants for which a variety of commercial reagents are available.
[b]Anti-Leu series are a product of Becton Dickenson (Mountain View, CA).
[c]OKT series are a product of Ortho Diagnostics (Raritan, NJ).
[d]W3/13, W3/25, and OX8 are distributed by Accurate Chemical.
[e]Reagents with specificity including but not limited to cells indicated.
[f]MAC-1 is available from Hybritech Inc. (San Diego) or Accurate Chemical (Westbury, NY).
[g]GM 1.2 is a product of New England Nuclear (Boston, MA).

At present, the routine analysis of hemopoietic stem cell populations is largely confined to the use of colony-forming assays that measure the clonal expansion of differentiated stem cell progeny (see chapters by E. P. Cronkite and F. D. Wilson, *this volume*). As a result, the early stages of differentiation from pluripotential stem cell to myeloid and erythroid cell lines are incompletely defined. Alternative methods that would enable the identification and sorting of bone marrow stem cell populations are actively being pursued in a number of laboratories. Van den Engh and co-workers have used the simultaneous measurement of low and right angle light scatter to crudely separate mouse bone marrow cells and to enrich colony-forming unit spleen (CFU-S) cells (52). Figure 2 illustrates the degree of resolution into erythrocyte, lymphocyte, blast, and myeloid populations that can currently be achieved using light scatter measurements alone. Sorting bone marrow cells on the basis of light scatter is not efficient enough for the separation of stem cells for transplantation, but in combination with physical separation techniques can improve the yield of stem cell populations (52).

Merocyanine 540 is a cationic dye with the exceptional property of being permeable only to cells with excitable membranes (15). This characteristic appears to be independent of membrane polarity and enables the discrimination of immature hemopoietic and leukemic cells from mature cell populations on the basis of staining with the compound (42,51). Figure 10 illustrates differences in merocyanine 540 staining between mature murine spleen cells and bone marrow cell populations, the latter containing a substantial number of early differentiating hemopoietic and progenitor cells.

A number of monoclonal antibodies have been partially characterized that exhibit some specificity toward stem cells. Results of these studies suggest antigenic heterogeneity in both CFU-S and CFU-granulocyte-macrophage (GM) cell populations. These results are entirely consistent with the heterogeneity previously observed in CFU assays and are discussed by Dr. Cronkite *(this volume)*. Such findings present the intriguing possibility that these antigenic differences may correspond to further discernable stages in stem cell differentiation. Beverley et al. (4) reported the production of two mouse monoclonal antibodies, one that

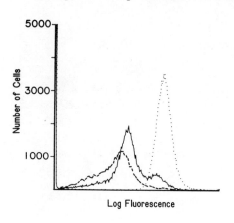

FIG. 10. Binding of merocyanine 540 to murine spleen, bone marrow, and malignant lymphoma cells. Normal murine spleen *(dashed line)*, bone marrow *(solid line)*, and RL-12NP cells *(dotted line)*.

appears specific for human myeloid cells and another that presumptively recognizes all bone marrow progenitor cells, including myeloid, erythroid, and lymphoid precursors. Similar results were reported by Bodger et al. (5) employing the simultaneous use of two monoclonal antibodies to isolate human pluripotent stem cells. Ferrero et al. (16) defined antigenically distinct subpopulations of myeloid progenitor cells present in human peripheral blood and bone marrow that were identified using mouse antilymphomonocytic monoclonal antibodies. Other investigators have reported the production of rat monoclonal antibodies directed against murine bone marrow cells that react with subpopulations of lymphocytes, granulocyte, and macrophage precursors but appear to be absent from erythroid cells (12,53). Recently, Harris et al. (21) provided preliminary characterization of a monoclonal antibody, Qa-m2, that recognizes a subset of murine CFU-S cells corresponding to the 14-day colonies described by Siminovitch et al. (47), the significance of which is discussed in detail in Dr. Cronkite's chapter. Such antigenic differences between subsets of hemopoietic stem cells may play a functional role in hemopoietic differentiation. Obviously, the availability of antigenic markers for quantitating and discriminating hemopoietic stem cells will greatly facilitate the evaluation of bone marrow toxicity and enable the study of subtle effects on stem cell homing and differentiation that can only be approached indirectly using colony-forming assay methods alone.

SUMMARY

Hematologic abnormalities resulting from exposure to toxic agents may occur as result of injury to or the death of the formed elements of the blood, damage to bone marrow stem cells, and/or interference with the maturation and development of the progenitors of circulating blood cells. Until recently, these events could only be examined indirectly, using relatively insensitive techniques that failed to resolve changes at the level of the individual cell. Presently, FCF technology provides the ability to measure a variety of parameters on individual cells. These include, but are not limited to, DNA, RNA, protein, enzyme activities, surface antigens, calcium flux, and plasma membrane potential. The application of these techniques in various combinations provides us with the opportunity to identify blood and bone marrow cells and to measure their individual proliferative status and functional characteristics.

Nowhere is the potential of FCF more evident than in the study of cell surface characteristics. Over the past decade recognition of the importance of the plasma membrane in the regulation of cell growth and differentiation has gained tremendous momentum. As discussed by Dr. Cronkite *(this volume)* all cells in the course of differentiation express an increased number and diversity of surface receptors that when bound by other cells or regulatory molecules, influence cell function and growth. Our knowledge of the nature and role of these surface antigens as expressed on hemopoietic cells is far from complete; however, these molecules not only provide us with a tool for identifying individual cell types but also can be correlated with cell proliferative status and function. We are thus afforded unparalleled sensitivity for the study of the regulation of cell growth and differentiation.

REFERENCES

1. Bagwell, C. B., Hudson, J. L., and Irvin, G. L. (1979): Nonparametric flow cytometry analysis. *J. Histochem. Cytochem.*, 27:293–296.
2. Barlogie, B., Drewinko, B., Schumann, J., Gohde, W., Dosik, G., Latreille, J., Johnston, D. A., and Freireich, E. J. (1980): Cellular DNA content as a marker of neoplasia in man. *Am. J. Med.*, 69:195–203.
3. Barlogie, B., Hittelman, W., Spitzer, G., Trujillo, J. M., Hart, J. S., Smallwood, L., and Drewinko, B. (1977): Correlation of DNA distribution abnormalities with cytogenetic findings in human adult leukemia and lymphoma. *Cancer Res.*, 37:440–447.
4. Beverley, P. C. L., Linch, D., and Delia, D. (1980): Isolation of human haematopoietic progenitor cells using monoclonal antibodies. *Nature*, 287:332–333.
5. Bodger, M. P., Izaguirre, C. A., Blacklock, H. A., and Hoffbrand, V. (1983): Surface antigenic determinants on human pluripotent and unipotent hematopoietic progenitor cells. *Blood*, 61:1006–1010.
6. Braunstein, J. D., Melamed, M. R., Darzynkiewicz, Z., Traganos, F., Sharpless, T., and Good, R. A. (1975): Quantitation of transformed lymphocytes by flow cytometry. *Clin. Immunol. Immunopathol.*, 4:209–215.
7. Brawn, R. J., Barker, C. R., Oesterle, A. D., Kelly, R. J., and Dandliker, W. B. (1975): An improved fluorescence probe cytotoxicity assay. *J. Immunol. Methods*, 9:7–26.
8. Cram, L. S., Ardnt-Jovin, D. J., Grimwade, B. G., and Jovin, T. M. (1979): Fluorescence polarization and pulse width analysis of chromosomes by a flow system. *J. Histochem. Cytochem.*, 27:445–453.
9. Dangl, J. L., Parks, D. R., Oi, V. T., and Herzenberg, L. A. (1982): Rapid isolation of cloned isotype switch variants using fluorescence activated cell sorting. *Cytometry*, 2:395–401.
10. Darzynkiewicz, Z., Sharpless, T., Staiano-Coico, L., and Melamed, M. R. (1980): Subcompartments of the G1 phase cell cycle detected by flow cytometry. *Proc. Natl. Acad. Sci. USA*, 77:6696–6699.
11. Darzynkiewicz, Z., Traganos, F., Sharpless, T., and Melamed, M. R. (1976): Lymphocyte stimulation: a rapid multiparameter analysis. *Proc. Natl. Acad. Sci. USA*, 73:2881–2884.
12. Davis, J. M., Kubler, A.-M., and Conscience, J.-F. (1983): MBM-1, a differentiation marker of mouse hemopoietic cells defined by a rat monoclonal antibody. *Exp. Hematol.*, 11:332–340.
13. Dean, P. N., and Jett, J. H. (1974): Mathematical analysis of DNA histograms derived from flow microfluorometry. *J. Cell Biol.*, 60:523–527.
14. Dolbeare, F. A., and Phares, W. (1979): Naphthol AS-Bl (7-bromo-3-hydroxy-2-naphthol-o-anisidine) phosphatase and naphthol AS-B1 beta-D-glucuronidase in Chinese hamster ovary cells: biochemical and flow cytometric studies. *J. Histochem. Cytochem.*, 27:120–124.
15. Easton, T. G., Valinsky, J. E., and Reich, E. (1978): Merocyanine 540 as a fluorescent probe of membranes: staining of electrically excitable cells. *Cell*, 13:475–486.
16. Ferrero, D., Broxmeyer, H. E., Pagliardi, G. L., Venuta, S., Lange, B., Pessano, S., and Rovera, G. (1983): Antigenically distinct subpopulations of myeloid progenitor cells (CFU-GM) in human peripheral blood and bone marrow. *Proc. Natl. Acad. Sci. USA*, 80:4114–4118.
17. Freeman, D. A., and Cressman, H. A. (1975): Evaluation of six fluorescent protein stains for use in flow microfluorometry. *Stain Technol.*, 50:279–284.
18. Fried, J. (1977): Analysis of deoxyribonucleic acid histograms from flow cytofluorometry. Estimation of the distribution of cells within S phase. *J. Histochem. Cytochem.*, 25:942–951.
19. Goubin, G., Goldman, D. S., Luce, J., Neiman, P. E., and Cooper, G. M. (1983): Molecular cloning and nucleotide sequence of a transforming gene detected by transfection of chicken B-cell lymphoma DNA. *Nature*, 302:114–119.
20. Gray, J. W., Peters, D., Merrill, J. T., Martin, R., and Van Dilla, M. A. (1979): Slit-scan flow cytometry of mammalian chromosomes. *J. Histochem. Cytochem.*, 27:441–444.
21. Harris, R. A., Hogarth, P. M., Wadeson, L. J., Collins, P., McKenzie, I. F. C., and Penington, D. G. (1984): An antigenic difference between cells forming early and late haematopoietic spleen colonies (CFU-S). *Nature*, 307:638–641.

22. Horan, P. K., and Kappler, J. W. (1977): Automated fluorescent analysis for cytotoxicity assays. *J. Immunol. Methods*, 18:309–316.
23. Horan, P. K., Muirhead, K. A., Gorton, S., and Irons, R. D. (1980): A rabbit bone marrow model system for the evaluation of cytotoxicity. Asceptic aspiration of bone marrow cells. *J. Lab. Anim. Sci.*, 30:76–79.
24. Hutter, K.-J., and Stohr, M. (1982): Rapid detection of mutagen induced micronucleated erythrocytes by flow cytometry. *Histochemistry*, 75:353–362.
25. Irons, R. D. (1981): Benzene-induced myelotoxicity: application of flow cytofluorometry for the evaluation of early proliferative change in bone marrow. *Environ. Health. Perspect.*, 39:39–49.
26. Irons, R. D., Heck, H. D'A., Moore, B. J., and Muirhead, K. A. (1979): Effects of short term benzene administration on bone marrow cell cycle kinetics in the rat. *Toxicol. Appl. Pharmacol.*, 51:399–409.
27. Irons, R. D., Stillman, W. S., and Dean, J. H. (1983): Application of flow cytometric methods in immunotoxicology. In: *Proceedings of the Thirteenth Conference on Environmental Toxicology*, pp. 24–32. Air Force Aerospace Medical Research Laboratory, Wright-Patterson Air Force Base, Ohio AFAMRL-TR-82-101.
28. Jovin, T. M. (1979): Fluorescence polarization and energy transfer: theory and application. In: *Flow Cytometry and Sorting*, edited by M. R. Melamed, P. F. Mullaney, and M. L. Mendelsohn, pp. 137–166, John Wiley & Sons, New York.
29. Judd, W., Poordry, C. A., and Strominger, J. L. (1980): Novel surface antigen expressed on dividing cells but absent from nondividing cells. *J. Exp. Med.*, 152:1430–1435.
30. Kreth, H. W., and Herzenberg, L. A. (1974): Fluorescence-activated cell sorting of human T and B lymphocytes. *Cell. Immunol.*, 12:396–406.
31. Kvaloy, S., Langholm, R., Kaalhus, O., Michaelsen, T., Funderud, S., Foss Abrahamsen, A., and Godal, T. (1984): Transferrin receptor and B-lymphoblast antigen—their relationship to DNA synthesis, histology and survival in B-cell lymphomas. *Intl. J. Cancer*, 33:173–177.
32. Larrick, J. W., and Cresswell, P. (1979): Transferrin receptors on human B and T lymphoblastoid cell lines. *Biochim. Biophys. Acta*, 583:483–490.
33. Latt, S. A. (1979): Fluorescent probes of DNA microstructure and synthesis. In: *Flow Cytometry and Sorting*, edited by M. R. Melamed, P. F. Mullaney, and M. L. Mendelsohn, pp. 263–284. John Wiley & Sons, New York.
34. Leary, J. F., Todd, P., Wood, J. C. S., and Jett, J. H. (1979): Laser flow cytometric light scatter and fluorescence pulse width and pulse rise-time sizing of mammalian cells. *J. Histochem. Cytochem.*, 27:315–320.
35. Lewis, J. G., and Swenberg, J. A. (1983): The kinetics of DNA alkylation, repair and replication in hepatocytes, Kupffer cells and sinusoidal endothelial cells in rat liver during continuous exposure to 1,2-dimethyl-hydrazine. *Carcinogenesis*, 4:529–536.
36. Linscott, W. D. (1984): Linscott's Directory of Immunological and Biological Reagents, 3rd ed. Linscott's Directory, Mill Valley, CA.
37. Madoc-Jones, H., and Mauro, F. (1974): Site of action of cytotoxic agents in the cell life cycle. In: *Antineoplastic and Immunosuppressive Agents*, Vol. 1. edited by A. C. Sartorelli and D. G. Johns, pp. 205–219. Springer-Verlag, New York.
38. Mauro, F., and Madoc-Jones, H. (1970): Age-responses of cultured mammalian cells to cytotoxic drugs. *Cancer Res.*, 30:1397–1408.
39. Miller, A. G. (1983): Ethylated fluoresceins: assay of cytochrome P-450 activity and application to measurements in single cells by flow cytometry. *Anal. Biochem.*, 133:46–57.
40. Muirhead, K. A., Irons, R. D., Bruins, R., and Horan, P. K. (1980): A rabbit bone marrow model system for the evaluation of cytotoxicity: characterization of normal bone marrow cell cycle parameters by flow cytometry. *Cytochemistry*, 28:526–532.
41. Rotman, B., and Papermaster, B. W. (1966): Membrane properties of living mammalian cells as studied by enzymatic hydrolysis of fluorogenic esters. *Proc. Natl. Acad. Sci. USA*, 55:134–141.
42. Schlegel, R. A., Phelps, B. M., Waggoner, A., Terada, L., and Williamson, P. (1980): Binding of merocyanine 540 to normal and leukemic erythroid cells. *Cell*, 20:321–328.
43. Schuette, W. H., Shackney, S. E., MacCollum, M. A., and Smith, C. A. (1983): High resolution method for the analysis of DNA histograms that is suitable for the detection of multiple aneuploid G1 peaks in clinical samples. *Cytometry*, 3:376–386.
44. Shapiro, H. M. (1981): Flow cytometric probes of early events in cell activation. *Cytometry*, 1:301–312.

45. Shapiro, H. M. (1983): Multistation multiparameter flow cytometry: a critical review and rationale. *Cytometry*, 3:227–243.
46. Sheck, L. E., Muirhead, K. A., and Horan, P. K. (1980): Evaluation of S phase distribution of flow cytometric DNA histograms by autoradiography and computer algorithms. *Cytometry*, 1:109–117.
47. Siminovitch, L., McCulloch, E. A., and Till, J. E. (1963): The distribution of colon-forming cells among spleen colonies. *J. Cell Comp. Physiol.*, 62:327–336.
48. Steinkamp, J. A., Wilson, J. S., Saunders, G. C., and Stewart, C. C. (1982): Phagocytosis: Flow cytometric quantitation with fluorescent microspheres. *Science*, 215:64–66.
49. Tanke, H. J., Nieuwenhuis, I. A. B., Koper, G. J. M., Slats, J. C. M., and Ploem, J. S. (1980): Flow cytometry of human reticulocytes based on RNA fluorescence. *Cytometry*, 1:313–320.
50. Traganos, F., Darzynkiewicz, Z., Sharpless, T., and Melamed, M. R. (1977): Simultaneous staining of ribonucleic acid and deoxyribonucleic acids in unfixed cells using acridine orange in a flow cytofluorometric system. *J. Histochem. Cytochem.*, 25:46–56.
51. Valinsky, J. E., Easton, T. G., and Reich, E. (1978): Merocyanine 540 as a fluorescent probe of membranes: selective staining of leukemic and immature hemopoietic cells. *Cell*, 13:487–499.
52. van den Engh, G., Visser, J., Bol, S., and Trask, B. (1980): Concentration of hemopoietic stem cells using a light-activated cell sorter. *Blood Cells*, 6:609–623.
53. Watt, S. M., Gilmore, D. J., Metcalf, D., Cobbold, S. P., Hoang, T. K., and Waldmann, H. (1983): Segregation of mouse hempoietic progenitor cells using the monoclonal antibody, YBM/42. *J. Cell Physiol.*, 115:37–45.
54. Wheeless, Jr., L. L. (1979): Slit-scanning and pulse width analysis. In: *Flow Cytometry and Sorting*, edited by M. R. Melamed, P. F. Mullaney, and M. L. Mendelsohn, pp. 125–135, John Wiley & Sons, New York.
55. Wofsy, L., and Henry, C. (1978): Hapten-sandwich labeling of cell-surface antigens. *Contemp. Top. Mol. Immunol.*, 7:215–237.

Toxicology of the Blood and Bone Marrow,
edited by Richard D. Irons. Raven Press,
New York © 1985. .

Cytogenetic Analysis of
Bone Marrow Damage

Raymond R. Tice and J. L. Ivett[1]

Medical Department, Brookhaven National Laboratory, Upton, New York 11973

The last decade has brought increased awareness of the sensitivity of the bone marrow to external and internal stimuli and, in particular, to the cytotoxic (i.e., damage to a cell which results in cell death) and/or genotoxic (i.e., damage to cellular DNA, which can cause cell death, mutations, cancer, etc.) effects of xenobiotic chemicals. As a result, considerable research has been devoted to developing *in vivo* bone marrow assays for detecting genotoxic damage induced by xenobiotics. First, the bone marrow is the major site of hematopoiesis and is comprised of several functionally distinct cell populations. Bone marrow damage can occur across cell lineages with all proliferating cell populations affected, or the damage can be relatively lineage and cell-type specific. Thus, effects on stem cells, proliferating cells, or differentiating cells can be assessed concurrently. Second, the high rate of cell turnover makes the bone marrow a sensitive target for carcinogenic/mutagenic chemicals. Its high mitotic rate and the ease of technical manipulation also make the bone marrow a favored experimental system of *in vivo* genetic toxicologists. Third, experimentally obtained data indicate the relevance of bone marrow damage to future adverse health effects. Cytotoxic damage to bone marrow cells can be easily related to diseases such as pancytopenia or anemia, and genotoxic damage can be correlated with tumor induction.

Cytogenetic manifestations of bone marrow damage, whether they be cytotoxic or genotoxic, provide unique opportunity for assessing events on a cell-by-cell basis. These manifestations include: (a) aneuploidy, (b) chromosomal aberrations, (c) micronuclei formation, (d) sister chromatid exchanges, and (e) alterations in cell cycle kinetics. With the exception of micronucleus evaluation, these cytogenetic endpoints require metaphase cells for evaluation, and, unfortunately, metaphase cells are generally not identifiable as to cell lineage. This restriction limits the usefulness of cytogenetic evaluations by not allowing a cell-type specific analysis of the induced response. Micronuclei, which can be selectively analyzed in specific cell types, can be used to assess the genotoxic effect of agents on cells of different lineages (e.g., leukocytes, erythrocytes).

---

[1]*Present address:* Litton Bionetics, Inc., Kensington, Maryland 20895

The purpose of this chapter is to discuss the biological basis for these various cytogenetic endpoints and their utility in assessing bone marrow damage. It will also be demonstrated that several of these independent measures of cytotoxic/ genotoxic damage can be integrated into one methodology offering increased resolution and sensitivity.

ANEUPLOIDY

Aneuploidy refers to alterations in chromosome number resulting from abnormal cytokinesis. The complete absence of normal disjunction during cell division results in the formation of polyploid cells (i.e., cells containing an even numbered multiple of the normal genome). Under some conditions, this process of polyploid formation occurs normally, as in the production of megakaryocytes (7). However, the loss or gain of one or a few chromosomes results in a genetic imbalance and the formation of abnormal cells. One theory of carcinogenesis is based on the imbalance of specific gene products resulting from chromosomal rearrangements and/or aneuploidy (17). In support of this theory, recent experimental data suggest that transformation, an *in vitro* process considered relevant to carcinogenesis, can be induced by aneugenic agents (3). Also, the induction in humans of chemotherapy-dependent secondary leukemias appears in some cases to involve the loss and/or gain of specific chromosomes (40). Thus, aneuploidy is a relevant genotoxic endpoint to assess in bone marrow cell populations.

The various mechanisms by which aneuploidy is induced are not well understood. The most commonly involved mechanism involves agent-induced interference with the spindle apparatus (66), which during anaphase acts to pull the segregating chromosomes to the poles. However, other mechanisms, including inactivation of the kinetochore and the centriole, cannot be excluded (66).

The ascertainment of aneuploid induction in bone marrow cells is not a trivial exercise and has been the focus of limited experimental research. The most common approach has involved collecting cells at metaphase using an appropriate spindle poison (e.g., colchicine, colcemid) and, after the routine cytological preparation of bone marrow material for microscopic evaluation, enumerating the number of chromosomes present in a suitable metaphase spread (13,22,28,46). However, this approach is often confounded by technical artifacts (e.g., chromosome loss due to cell breakage) associated with the cytological preparation of bone marrow tissue. These artifacts can lead to erroneously high frequencies of aneuploid cells (13,22).

Several modifications of the basic approach have been used in an attempt to circumvent various technical artifacts. For example, in statistically analyzing aneuploid frequency data, Liang et al. (28,46) utilized data only on the frequency of hyperploid cells. This discrimination between cells with greater than the normal chromosomal complement and those with less than the normal complement is based on the supposition that the technical artifacts associated with tissue processing and slide preparation can only lead to a loss of a chromosome(s) from a metaphase spread. Hyperploid metaphase spreads are assumed to result only from true aneuploid-inducing events. In support of this approach, vinblastine and colcemid, two well-known spindle poisons, induce a dose-dependent increase in hyperploid cells in mouse bone marrow (46). However a false gain in chromosome number, one that is not always identifiable by a discordant morphology between the additional chromosome(s) and the normal chromosome complement, can also result from technical manipulations. A chromosome lost by cell breakage from one metaphase spread can end up within a second metaphase spread and be considered as part of the normal complement. In addition, restricting the ascertainment to hyperploid cells limits the sensitivity of the methodology because, although all hyperploid cells also have a sister cell that is hypoploid, the reverse is not true. Lagging chromosomes can be omitted from either daughter cell, giving rise to a euploid and a hypoploid metaphase spread at the next division.

Another cytogenetic approach for identifying aneuploid bone marrow cells is based on identifying the posttreatment replicative history of individual metaphase cells (22). The replicative history is defined as the number of cell cycles (i.e., one, two, or three and more) completed in the presence of a heavy atom analog of thymidine, such as 5-bromodeoxyuridine (BrdUrd) (Fig. 1). Using this technique, the frequency of aneuploid cells (hypoploid and hyperploid) among first-generation, posttreatment metaphase spreads is compared with the aneuploid frequency among second-generation, posttreatment metaphase spreads. The usefulness of this comparison is based on the assumption that an aneuploid event requires cytokinesis and, consequently, that the frequency of aneuploid first-generation, posttreatment metaphase cells reflects technical manipulation and baseline frequencies whereas the frequency of aneuploid second-generation, posttreatment metaphase cells reflects technical artifact, baseline frequencies, and treatment-induced events. The effect of technical artifacts can be further reduced by analyzing both cell populations on the same microscope slide.

This approach has been used to assess the ability of diethylstilbestrol-diphosphate (DES-dp), a human carcinogen with suspected aneugenic properties (48), to induce aneuploid cells in the bone marrow of C57B1/6 mice (22). No significant differences in aneuploid frequencies between first-generation and second generation-metaphase cells were observed in either male or female mice treated with 100 mg/kg DES-dp (Table 1). However, data obtained with this method can be confounded by an inability to distinguish between cells that have completed $G_2 + M + G_1 + S + G_2 + M$ and those that have completed $G_1 + S + G_2 + M$. Thus, the first-generation, posttreatment metaphase cell population may have been contaminated with cells that had undergone cytokinesis after the onset of the treatment (i.e., they could be true aneuploid cells). Analysis of the timing of these events suggests that judicious application of agent treatment in relationship to the onset of BrdUrd exposure can significantly decrease the likelihood of the occurrence of these cells.

Both of these cytogenetic approaches require considerable validation before they can be applied routinely to the investigation of aneuploid induction in bone marrow. It may well be useful to integrate segments of these two approaches into one method

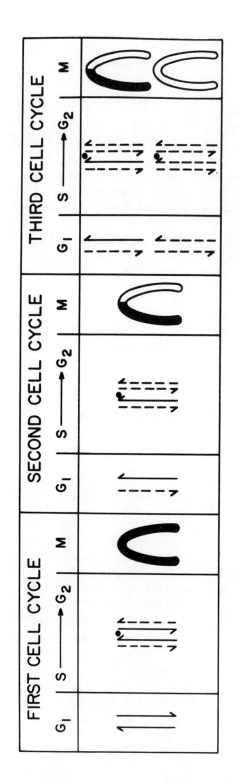

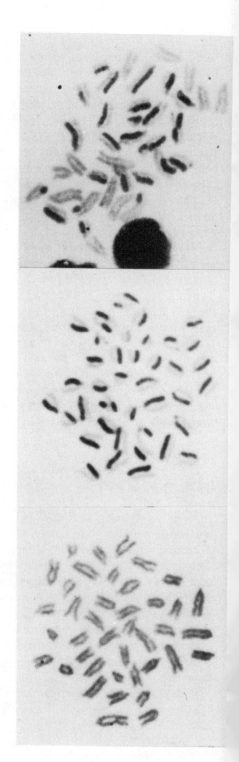

TABLE 1. Percent aneuploid cells
among first- and second-generation
metaphase cells in bone marrow of
DES-dp treated C67Bl/6 mice

	Cell generation	
Sex[a]	First[b]	Second[b]
Male	10.8 ± 2.2	12.8 ± 1.8
Female	17.2 ± 2.6	17.6 ± 2.0

[a]Randomized groups of mice (5/sex) were in-jected with DES-dp intraperitoneally at a dose of 100 mg/kg body weight 1 hr after the onset of BrdUrd infusion. Animals were killed 25 hr later [following a 2-hr treatment with demecol-cine (Colcemid)], the bone marrow was pro-cessed, and slides prepared. For each animal the chromosome complement of 50 first- and 50-second generation metaphase cells was determined (see ref. 22 for additional details).

[b]Mean percent aneuploid cells per animal ± SEM among animals.

offering increased sensitivity and reliability. Currently, two other approaches—micronucleus evaluation and flow microfluoremetric analysis (FMF)—can also be applied to the investigation of aneuploid induction. Micronucleus evaluation will be discussed in a later section of this chapter. In FMF analysis (see R. D. Irons and W. S. Stillman, *this volume*), the relative proportions of cells in different stages of the cell cycle ($G_1, S, G_2 + M$) are determined by measuring cellular DNA content (18,25). The coefficient of variation around the G_1 and the $G_2 + M$ peaks may be a useful indicator of the presence of aneuploid cells. Future studies will be necessary to investigate the possible application of this technique to aneuploid studies.

CHROMOSOMAL ABERRATIONS

Chromosomal aberrations (CAs) are broadly defined as alterations in chromosome morphology (Fig. 2). These alterations are usually assessed in cells at metaphase, but certain kinds of damage can also be detected during anaphase (e.g., anaphase bridges) or at interphase (micronuclei). Aberrations that involve identical positions on both sister chromatids of a chromosome are referred to as chromosome type, whereas those that involve only one of the two sister chromatids are referred to as chromatid-type. Within these two types, CAs may be further classified as (a) achromatic lesions or gaps, pale-staining chromatic regions apparently not involving a physical discontinuity or displacement of genetic material; (b) breaks or deletions,

FIG. 1. The incorporation of BrdUrd into DNA for three consecutive cell generations and a photomicrograph of corresponding fluorescence-plus-Giemsa stained, mouse bone marrow metaphase cell. Solid line, native DNA; dashed line, BrdUrd containing DNA.

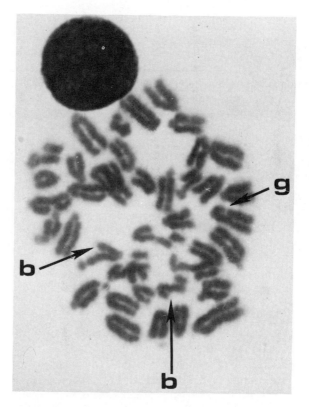

FIG. 2. Chromatid-type chromosomal aberrations induced by mitomycin C in first-generation posttreatment bone marrow cells of a B6C3F1 male mouse. *Arrows* indicate specific aberrations. g, gap; b, break.

physical discontinuities, and displacements of genetic material; and (c) rearrangements or exchanges, the exchange of genetic material within (intrachange) or between (interchange) chromosomes.

Most CAs are deleterious and result in cell death. However, some types (e.g., reciprocal translocations, small deletions, inversions) can lead to altered gene function(s) without an accompanying loss in cell viability. Alterations in gene function occurring as a result of interchanges between specific chromosome regions are correlated with the appearance of several different kinds of cancers (36), indicating the probable involvement of CAs in carcinogenesis. Consistent with this relationship, CAs are induced by many known mutagens and/or carcinogens (42). These findings make CA analysis a useful indicator of genotoxic and cytotoxic damage in bone marrow cells following *in vivo* exposures to xenobiotics.

Most mutagenic/carcinogenic chemicals induce CAs only when an intervening round of DNA replication occurs between the induction of DNA damage and the time of metaphase/anaphase/interphase analysis (16,42). Most, if not all, of the resulting chromosomal damage is of the chromatid-type (4,5,16,42,47). This dependency on DNA synthesis for the expression of CAs has led to the hypothesis that these aberrations occur as the result of DNA replication on a damaged template (5,16). Agents requiring DNA replication for the expression of clastogenic damage (i.e., chromosomal aberrations) are termed S-dependent. Conversely, agents like ionizing radiation and "radiomimetic" chemicals (e.g., bleomycin) that induce CAs without involving DNA synthesis are described as S-independent. This S-independency of formation leads to the induction of chromosome-type aberrations when cells are exposed to a DNA-damaging agent prior to S phase and to the formation of chromatid-type aberrations when cells are treated in S phase or G_2 (4,5,15,47). These two independent mechanisms for aberration formation have been interpreted to indicate that the formation of S-independent CAs involves DNA base damage whereas the formation of S-independent CAs involves DNA strand scissions (4,5,42,69).

Regardless of the mechanisms involved in the induction of the clastogenic damage, the presence of induced CAs in bone marrow cells indicates a cytotoxic/genotoxic health risk (e.g., anemia, leukemia). The magnitude and peak appearance of the clastogenic response in the bone marrow following an acute exposure to a genotoxic chemical depends on clastogenic mechanism, potency, dose, pharmacokinetics, and extent of cell proliferative inhibition. In metaphase or anaphase analysis, the maximum response is generally observed at a sample time that permits one round of DNA replication after the maximum induction of DNA damage. The maximal expression occurs at this time because, in the absence of chronic exposure conditions, further cell divisions lead to (a) a decline in CA frequency due to the dilution of CAs among daughter cells and (b) the selective loss of heavily damaged cells from the proliferating cell population. Since DNA damage can increase cell cycle duration, CA testing protocols (e.g., ref. 42) require multiple sampling times (i.e., at 6, 24, and 48 hours after an acute exposure treatment).

An alternative approach to multiple sampling involves the use of the BrdUrd-dependent differential staining technique already discussed (21,22,33,62). This technique permits the unequivocal identification of metaphase cells that have completed one and only one round of DNA replication since the onset of BrdUrd exposure. By appropriate timing of agent treatment in relationship to BrdUrd exposure, metaphase cells that offer an optimal opportunity for the expression of clastogenic damage can be selected. This approach has recently undergone extensive validation under the auspices of the U.S. National Toxicology Program (refs. 21,33,62; see section on "Cell Cycle Analysis"). The ability to identify the replicative history of individual metaphase cells and to collect data from bone marrow sampled at optimal times offer increased sensitivity at a reduced effort. The only inherent confounding factor is the possible synergistic or antagonistic interaction between the test compound and the BrdUrd-containing DNA (56). The probability of this interaction can be minimized by exposing the bone marrow cells to the test agent prior to BrdUrd incorporation into cellular DNA. A limited analysis (mitomycin C, dimethylbenzanthracene, and cyclophosphamide) of CAs induced in bone marrow cells of animals with and without exposure to BrdUrd supports the validity of this approach (32) (Table 2).

MICRONUCLEI

As indicated earlier (see section on "Chromosomal Aberrations"), micronuclei (MN) are cytoplasmic nuclear bodies that occur as a result of the exclusion of acentric chromosomal fragments or lagging chromosomes from daughter nuclei during cytokinesis (reviewed in refs. 20,51). Because of the speed and simplicity involved in MN identification, MN analysis is often used as a sensitive, yet less expensive and less time-consuming alternative to classical metaphase analysis (20). As with all cytogenetic endpoints, MN formation requires cell division. However, as opposed to CAs, sister chromatid exchange and cell kinetic analysis, scoring of MN does not depend on metaphase preparations but is determined in interphase cells.

Although several forms of MN assessment have been developed, the best developed and most pertinent form of MN evaluation involves the scoring of MN in bone marrow polychromatic erythrocytes (PCEs) (reviewed in ref. 20). The product of recent cell divisions, these anucleated cells are fully differentiated, abundant, and easily recognized. In addition, they have a residency time in the bone marrow of approximately 24 hours, and exhibit a low spontaneous background of MN (20). Thus, analysis of MN in PCEs provides information about recent bone marrow clastogenic or aneugenic damage.

As would be expected, there is a strong concordance between CA-inducing and MN-inducing agents. The fact that MN can also arise through a mechanism independent of direct DNA damage is both an important attribute and a confounding factor. MN evaluation is one of few methods useful for the detection of aneuploid events in a differentiating cell line. Yet, the inability to readily distinguish between clastogenic- and aneugenic-produced MN makes the mechanistic interpretation of

TABLE 2. *Frequency of bone marrow CAs induced by mitomycin C in B6C3F1 male mice with and without a concurrent exposure to BrdUrd[a]*

MMC (mg/kg)	With BrdUrd			Without BrdUrd		
	Events/cell[b]	% Damaged cells[c]	N	Events/cell[b]	% Damaged cells[c]	N
0	0.034 ± 0.009	5.0 ± 0.8	5	0.023 ± 0.009	2.1 ± 0.8	7
2.5	0.160 ± 0.025	10.3 ± 1.7	3	0.145 ± 0.025	9.5 ± 0.5	2
4.0	0.310 ± 0.040	16.5 ± 2.2	4	0.240 ± 0.058	12.7 ± 1.2	3
10.0	0.750 ± 0.026	38.3 ± 3.4	4	0.953 ± 0.040	25.2 ± 3.8	4

[a]All animals were infused with BrdUrd for 10 hr. Intraperitoneal (i.p.) injection of mitomycin C (MMC) occurred 1 hr after initiation of infusion. Demecolcine (Colcemid) was injected (i.p.) into each animal 2 hr prior to bone marrow sampling. One hundred first-generation metaphase cells were analysed per animal. (See refs. 54 and 61 for additional technical details.)
[b]Group mean number of breakage events (including gaps) per cell ± SEM between N animals.
[c]Group mean percent metaphase cells with aberrations (including gaps) ± SEM between N animals.

MN data extremely difficult. Several approaches have been considered for the identification of micronuclei origin. For example, aneugenically induced MN are generally larger than clastogenically induced MN (72). However, considerable overlap in size and/or DNA content can be expected to occur between MN induced by these two independent mechanisms, making an identification of the origin of individual MN somewhat equivocal. The discovery of antibodies against chromosome kinetochore regions (9) offers the possibility of a more definitive method for identifying MN origin. Clastogenic-induced MN would not contain a kinetochore, whereas aneugenic-induced MN could.

As with any cytogenetic evaluation of bone marrow genotoxic damage, the timing of sample collection in relation to treatment is an important parameter to consider in MN analysis. The optimal bone marrow sampling time for micronucleated PCEs depends on the mechanism of action, pharmacokinetic considerations, and the extent of suppression of PCE production (20). Because of agent-specific effects on bone marrow proliferation, multiple sampling times between 24 and 72 hours are recommended in order to avoid a false-negative result (20). This dependency of expression on bone marrow kinetics, the inability to distinguish between aneugenic- and clastogenic-induced MN, and the restriction of the assay to acute exposure protocols are the main limitations of evaluating bone marrow micronucleated PCEs.

A variation of micronucleated PCE analysis in the mouse offers increased simplicity and sensitivity while avoiding many of the constraints involved in assessing MN in bone marrow tissue. It is based on assessing MN in PCEs and in normochromatic erythrocytes (NCEs) of the peripheral blood (Fig. 3; refs. 31,49,63). Analyzing MN frequency in peripheral blood cells permits multiple sampling from the same animal under chronic or acute exposure conditions and an ascertainment of both recent and past bone marrow damage. This latter advantage is based on the fact that PCEs have a lifetime of 1 to 2 days in the peripheral blood and thus can indicate damage induced in the bone marrow 1 to 3 days prior to sampling and that NCEs in the mouse have a lifetime of 35 to 50 days in the peripheral blood and thus can be used to indicate damage induced in bone marrow over that time period (31,49,63).

Analysis of MN in mouse peripheral blood erythrocytes has proven to be an exceedingly useful technique for investigating time-dependent bone marrow sensitivity to the cytotoxic/genotoxic action of mutagens/carcinogens. For example, we have been able to demonstrate that (a) benzene at ambient concentrations as low as 10 ppm for 6 hours per day for 9 days induces a significant increase in MN in peripheral blood erythrocytes (Table 3, ref. 63); (b) benzene induces less damage in bone marrow cells at 16 weeks of exposure than at 8 weeks of exposure; (c) intermittent treatment with hydroquinone and phenol, two metabolites of benzene, are more damaging to bone marrow cells than are chronic treatments at the same dose (R. Tice and R. Irons, *unpublished data*); and (d) acute exposure to radiation induces bone marrow damage expressed in PCEs 7 days posttreatment, suggesting the presence of residual bone marrow damage (35). The results of these initial experiments clearly indicate that peripheral blood MN analysis can contribute

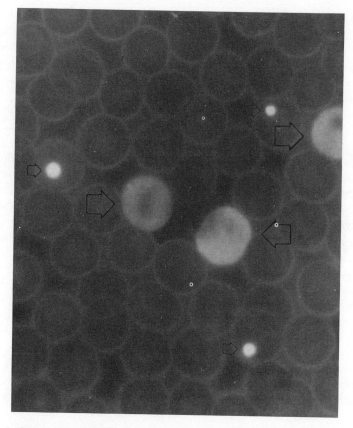

FIG. 3. Acridine-orange (AO)-stained mouse peripheral blood smear. Large *arrows* indicate PCEs (stained red with AO), small *arrows* indicate MN (stained yellow with AO), other cells are NCEs.

significantly to our understanding of hematopoiesis under chronic exposure conditions.

Unfortunately, the peripheral blood MN test cannot be used in all species. In humans (6), rats (50), and the white-footed mouse (30), the spleen removes circulating micronucleated erythrocytes; in the house mouse (31) and in the Syrian golden hamster (39), micronucleated erythrocytes persist in the peripheral blood. This species difference limits the widespread utility of this method.

One possible future advantage of the bone marrow/peripheral blood MN assay over other cytogenetic assays is the potential for interface with FMF techniques. Using a nucleic acid-specific stain such as acridine orange would allow identification of MN and PCEs, providing a time-dependent analysis of MN formation and expression. The versatility and usefulness of FMF-coupled MN evaluation is an extremely important research area requiring further investigation.

TABLE 3. *Induction of MN in the peripheral blood erythrocytes of C57Bl/6 male mice exposed to benzene 6 hr/day for 9 days[a]*

Benzene (ppm)	MN/PCE[b]	MN/NCE[b]	% PCE[c]	N
0	4.0 ± 0.4	3.9 ± 0.3	2.1 ± 0.1	20
10	4.4 ± 0.6	7.0 ± 0.4[d]	2.1 ± 0.1	10
25	7.3 ± 0.9[d]	6.5 ± 0.4[d]	2.3 ± 0.2	20
100	18.2 ± 1.5[d]	7.6 ± 0.6[d]	2.6 ± 0.4	20
400	21.7 ± 2.6	14.3 ± 1.7[d]	3.2 ± 0.4	10

[a]Blood smears were prepared from each animal 1 day after the last exposure, stained with acridine orange, and examined using epi-illuminated fluorescence microscopy. Data from two independent experiments are combined (63).

[b]Group mean number of micronuclei per 1,000 PCEs or 1,000 NCEs ± SEM among N animals.

[c]Group mean percent PCE in 1,000 erythrocytes ± SEM among N animals.

[d]Significantly different from control values by the Mann-Whitney U-test at $p < .05$.

SISTER CHROMATID EXCHANGE

Sister chromatid exchange (SCE) formation involves the breakage of and rejoining between the two DNA duplexes (one in each sister chromatid) present in a eukaryote chromosome after the completion of DNA replication (Fig. 4, reviewed in refs. 44,59,60,70). SCEs are primarily elicited in response to DNA synthetic activity on a damaged template (57,71), the magnitude of the response being proportional to the level of DNA damage (1,29,41,43,58). In the absence of cell lethality, the exact number of SCEs elicited by any DNA-damaging treatment depends on (a) the nature (1,29,41,43,58) and the genomic distribution (11,55) of the pertinent DNA lesion(s), (b) the efficiency of the appropriate DNA repair system in removing the lesion(s) (45,57,64), and (c) the temporal relationship between the formation of the primary DNA damage and the onset of scheduled DNA synthesis in the presence of BrdUrd (e.g., refs. 45,57). The incorporation of BrdUrd or some other heavy analog of thymidine into DNA for one or two cell cycles is necessary for the visualization of SCEs in second-generation metaphase cells (56).

Not all classes of genotoxic agents are equally capable of inducing SCEs. S-independent clastogenic agents such as ionizing radiation and radiomimetic chemicals (see section on CAs) are poor inducers of SCEs (29,41,58). On the other hand, S-dependent agents, which primarily cause DNA base damage, typically elicit a good SCE response (1,29,41,43,58). Antimetabolites can also induce SCEs, but the magnitude of the response is generally weak (19,58).

Unfortunately, the exact nature of the lesion(s), as well as the molecular events involved in SCE formation, remain unresolved. It has been suggested that the primary lesion (see refs. 57,69) is a DNA-DNA cross-link or a specific alkylation product [e.g., 3-adenine (38)]. However, since UV-light-induced pyrimidine dimers

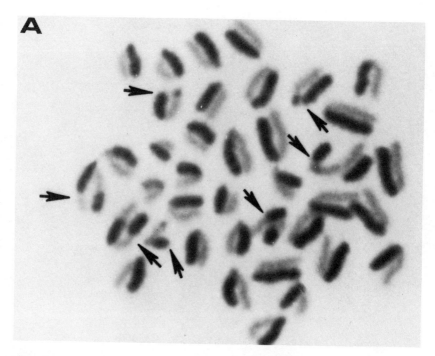

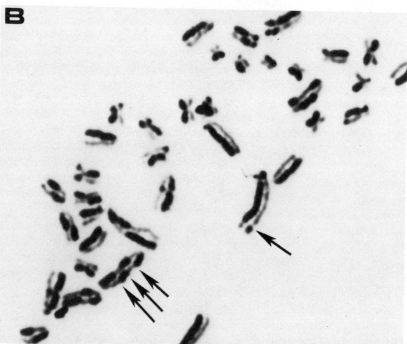

FIG. 4. Fluorescence-plus-Giemsa-stained, second-generation bone marrow cells. **A:** Metaphase cell from a control B6C3F1 mouse. **B:** Metaphase cell from a Sprague-Dawley rat treated with mitomycin C. *Arrows* indicate all of the SCEs present in the control cell and some of the SCEs present in the treated cell.

(43), alkylating agents and intercalaters all induce SCEs (1,29,41,43,58), it is quite likely that more than one kind of lesion is capable of eliciting an SCE response. Moreover, the observation that SCEs are also induced by treatments that do not appear to cause direct DNA damage [e.g., antimetabolites (19,58)] suggests that there may be more than one biological process capable of eliciting an SCE response. The SCE formation is limited to the S phase of the cell cycle, and since fixation of mutational events also appears to require DNA replication, some investigators have speculated that SCEs represent a cytological manifestation of a mutational event (i.e., an error-prone process). However, attempts to verify this hypothesis have resulted in conflicting data (10). Several compounds exist that are capable of inducing high levels of SCE but that apparently do not induce mutations (8). Thus, at least some SCEs are not associated with a mutagenic process.

The usefulness of assessing SCEs in bone marrow cells is based on their being sensitive indicators of genotoxic damage (see above) and their ease of scoring. For many genotoxic agents the frequency of SCEs is significantly increased after exposure to concentrations not associated with an increase in the frequency of chromosomal aberrations (41,58). Furthermore, only one-half to one-fourth as many metaphase cells must typically be examined for adequate statistical analysis in SCE studies (67), as compared with CA analysis (68). Thus, SCE assessment generally provides greater sensitivity than CA analysis for assessing the potential of agents to damage DNA in addition to a considerable savings in time and effort.

Several independent approaches have been developed for ensuring adequate incorporation of BrdUrd for at least one round of DNA replication within bone marrow cells. The most useful techniques include multiple intraperitoneal injections (27), subcutaneous implantation of a BrdUrd tablet (2), and continuous intravenous infusion of a BrdUrd isotonic solution (54). The first two BrdUrd delivery systems produce similar BrdUrd conditions *in vivo*, assuring an adequate supply of BrdUrd to the bone marrow for approximately 12 hours. However, the 12-hour period limits the flexibility of bone marrow SCE analysis because the first S phase must occur within this interval. Cells that have not completed one full round and only one round of DNA replication will exhibit discontinuous differential labeling patterns. Although both techniques offer technical simplicity, the 7 to 10 hourly injections required for the multiple-injection technique necessitates extensive animal handling. Pellet implantation, on the other hand, requires minor surgery and, thus, light anesthesia. Both procedures, however, leave the animals unrestrained throughout the duration of the experiment.

Continuous infusion of BrdUrd is technically more difficult and places the animal in a restrained condition. However, animals can be exposed to BrdUrd for as long as is considered necessary, thereby ensuring that regardless of the extent of cell division delay, BrdUrd will be present for incorporation into newly synthesized DNA for the required number of cell generations. Thus, this approach offers the greatest flexibility for SCE assessment in various animal tissues with different cell replicative rates or in tissues proliferating slower than normal owing to cytostatic effects. Recently, several techniques have been developed that greatly strengthen the utility of the pellet implantation method. Coating the pellet completely with agar (24) or partially with paraffin (32) extends BrdUrd availability to approximately 30 hours. This extended availability circumvents the main limitation associated with the pellet implantation method and makes this technique the method of choice.

The statistical requirements for analyzing SCEs in bone marrow cells have been examined and it was concluded that 25 cells per animal with 3 to 5 animals per data point provide an adequate *in vivo* sample size (67). Furthermore, since SCEs are scored in a defined cell population (i.e., in second-generation metaphase cells), multiple sampling times are not required. The main technical problems associated with this bioassay is that BrdUrd alters the rate of cell proliferation (see section on "Cell Cycle Analysis") and induces SCEs (reviewed in ref. 56). There is also some evidence to suggest that BrdUrd-substituted DNA may have an altered sensitivity to some chemicals (reviewed in ref. 56). However, these difficulties can be easily overcome through the inclusions of appropriate experimental controls and judicious agent treatment to BrdUrd exposure timing.

Recent research supported by the National Toxicology Program has investigated the optimal timing of exposure to toxic agent versus BrdUrd treatment, as well as the sampling time constraints involved in the mouse bone marrow bioassay (33,62). Based on the data obtained in these studies, the maximal yield of SCEs was agent-dependent and dependent on the time of injection of the test agent in relationship to the onset of BrdUrd treatment. Nevertheless, all time intervals resulted in a positive SCE response. Consequently, because of concerns about a possible synergistic interaction between BrdUrd-substituted DNA and the test compound and to limit handling of carcinogen-treated animals, injecting the test chemical within an hour after the onset of BrdUrd administration was considered advisable (62). Also, because the induced SCE frequency among early, mid, and late second-generation metaphase cells remained relatively constant, it was concluded that the time for sampling second-generation bone marrow metaphase cells was not critical (34).

The strengths of SCE analysis in bone marrow cells include the sensitivity of the endpoint to chemicals that produce DNA base damage, the ease and rapidity with which a bone marrow sample can be analyzed, and the use of BrdUrd incorporation to define cell kinetics (see following section). The limitations include insensitivity to agents inducing only DNA strand breakage, the unknown mechanism(s) involved in SCE formation, and the potential interaction between BrdUrd-substituted DNA and the test chemical.

CELL CYCLE ANALYSIS

Analysis of cellular kinetics in bone marrow cell populations has become useful as an indicator of alterations in hematopoiesis induced by internal and external signals or by exposure to xenobiotics. Historically, cell cycle duration has most often been determined using tritiated thymidine labeling (reviewed in ref. 12).

However, this technique is time consuming and suffers from technical and interpretive limitations (e.g., ref. 37), precluding its routine use in the assessment of bone marrow kinetics. During the last decade, two additional methods, FMF analysis and BrdUrd-dependent replicative history analysis, have been developed which are more suited for analyzing bone marrow cellular kinetics. FMF analysis (see chapter by R. D. Irons and W. S. Stillman, *this volume*) compares the relative proportions of cells in different stages of the cell cycle (i.e., G_1, S, $G_2 + M$) by measuring cellular DNA content (18,25). Alterations in these proportions are used to assess agent-induced or physiologically induced effects on cell cycle kinetics. Standard FMF analysis is limited in that (a) the replicative history of individual cells cannot be determined, (b) there is a requirement for single-cell suspensions, and (c) there is considerable equipment expense.

Analysis of BrdUrd-dependent differentially stained metaphase cells is, for some purposes, a more useful technique than FMF analysis for routine monitoring of bone marrow kinetics. This technique, already discussed in the preceding sections, allows an unequivocal identification of the number of S phases (and thus cell cycles) completed during bone marrow exposure to BrdUrd (23,60). Although originally developed for the visualization of DNA replication kinetics (26) and SCEs (see section on "Sister Chromatid Exchanges"), this technique has been adapted to the microscopic analysis of cell cycle kinetics. Using the differential staining patterns (Fig. 1), individual metaphase cells are identified as to the number of rounds of DNA replications (one, two, three, etc.) completed in the presence of BrdUrd (23,60). Bone marrow data obtained in this fashion can be analyzed (a) by comparing the relative proportions of metaphase cells with different replicative histories (22,61,62); (b) by calculating a replicative index (RI; ref. 52), a derived index that reflects the relative contribution of each cell cycle to the sampled population; and (c) by average generation time (AGT) analysis (23), a method that utilizes RI data in a time-dependent manner.

AGT analysis is ideally suited for the analysis of cell cycle kinetics in bone marrow and is calculated as follows:

$$AGT \ (hr) = \frac{\text{hours since onset of BrdUrd exposure}}{RI}$$

where the RI = (1 × frequency of first-generation metaphase cells)
+ (2 × frequency of second-generation metaphase cells)
+ (3 × frequency of third-generation metaphase cells)
+ ...

Lacking an ability to adequately differentiate between third- and subsequent generation metaphase cells, AGT analysis is limited to termination times where fourth-generation cells are nonexistent. Also, the presence of only first-generation metaphase cells will lead to a serious underestimation of the true AGT.

In Table 4, DES-dp-induced alterations in bone marrow kinetics are presented using the various methods for BrdUrd-dependent replicative history analysis. As

TABLE 4. *Inhibition of mouse (female C57Bl/6) bone marrow cellular proliferation by DES-dp*

Dose		Percent				
(mg/kg)	N	First[a]	Second[a]	Third[a]	RI[a]	AGT (hr)[a]
0	5	11.8 ± 4.2	79.2 ± 3.8	9.0 ± 2.8	1.97 ± 0.06	13.2 ± 0.05
5	6	16.0 ± 4.3	70.3 ± 2.1	13.7 ± 3.4	1.98 ± 0.10	13.1 ± 0.5
10	6	26.5 ± 8.8	67.2 ± 6.8	6.3 ± 3.5	1.80 ± 0.12	14.4 ± 1.0
25	11	32.4 ± 6.0	61.0 ± 4.8	5.6 ± 3.2	1.71 ± 0.08	15.2 ± 0.7
50	8	55.4 ± 11.0	41.4 ± 9.9	3.2 ± 2.3	1.48 ± 0.11	17.6 ± 1.5

All animals were injected intraperitoneally with DES-dp 1 hr after the onset of BrdUrd infusion and killed 25 hr later (see text, Table 1 and ref. 22 for additional details). One hundred randomly selected metaphase cells were identified as to the number of cell cycles completed since the onset of BrdUrd infusion.

[a]Mean value per animal ± SEM between N animals. RI, replicative index; AGT, average generation time.

can be seen, AGT analysis offers the simplest approach for analyzing the data. The bone marrow cells in this study were collected from animals killed after the same BrdUrd exposure period. However, samples obtained after different BrdUrd exposure periods can also be used in this method. The dose of BrdUrd used in these studies significantly delayed bone marrow proliferation kinetics (53). However, when assuming agent-induced delays, the BrdUrd-induced delay is unimportant, as appropriate controls are always incorporated in any study. If AGT analysis is being conducted to examine *de novo* bone marrow cell cycle kinetics, a BrdUrd dose-response curve must be obtained to ensure the use of a noninhibitory concentration of BrdUrd (53,54).

Statistical analysis of cell cycle kinetics by AGT, although advantageous when compared with the other approaches, is not without inherent limitations. First, AGT is a mean value derived from measurements on a sample of cells assumed to be homogenous with respect to their proliferative rate reflecting the replicative dynamics of the bone marrow in general. However, the accuracy of AGT analysis is potentially limited by several factors—one inherent to the scoring procedure and the other based on limitations associated with differential staining techniques. In the analysis of the replicative history of individual metaphase cells, only integer cell cycles are recorded. Noninteger labeling patterns observed in metaphase cells that have already entered S phase before BrdUrd becomes available for incorporation into the DNA are not distinguished from integer labeling patterns. Also, since the labeling patterns are based on the incorporation of BrdUrd into replicating DNA, it is not possible to distinguish between metaphase cells that have only progressed through one S phase (i.e., $S + G_2 + M$) and those that have additionally progressed through one complete cell cycle plus part of another (i.e., $G_2 + M + G_1 + S + G_2 + M$). Although both factors may alter the AGT, their impact on AGT analysis should cancel each other and the calculated AGT will not differ significantly from the true cell cycle duration.

A second, more profound limitation is that AGT analysis assumes that any alterations in the cell cycle is uniformly distributed over all cell generations. However, since the greatest proportions of cells examined have usually progressed through only one or two replications, the effect of cell generation specific cell cycle alterations should be minimized.

Third, genotoxic effects or sampling times that result in finding only first-generation metaphase cells cannot be included in AGT analysis. Without the presence of second-generation metaphase cells it is impossible to accurately calculate AGT values.

Finally, AGT analysis is dependent on logarithmic growth conditions. Cells undergoing proliferative stimulation with growth factors cannot be used in calculating AGT values until logarithmic growth is attained.

Nevertheless, the AGT methodology for analyzing bone marrow (and other tissue) kinetics has several advantages over other BrdUrd methods for analyzing cell kinetic rates. The calculated AGT is in hours and thus directly corresponds to the cell cycle time. AGT analysis incorporates all replicative history data, providing for greater sensitivity in detecting true alterations in the rate of cell cycle kinetics. Also, AGT analysis is largely independent of sample collection time. This system is technically simple and does not require great expertise or expensive equipment. Finally, AGT analysis has the potential for being used in conjunction with FMF techniques (e.g., ref. 14; see R. D. Irons and W. S. Stillman, *this volume*).

DISCUSSION

The various cytogenetic endpoints—aneuploidy, chromosomal aberrations, micronuclei, sister chromatid exchanges, cell cycle kinetics—discussed here are useful in assessing cytotoxic/genotoxic damage to bone marrow cells. However, with the exception of micronucleus analysis, it is impossible to identify the functional nature of the metaphase cell being examined for manifestations of damage. Thus, it is difficult to conclude whether all bone marrow elements are equally affected and/or are equally sensitive to the action of a xenobiotic chemical or physiological abnormality. Only with micronucleus analysis can the functional lineage (e.g., erythrocytic) of the affected cell be determined. This merging of functionally distinct cell populations into one "homogeneous" sample is the single major limitation associated with the cytogenetic evaluation of bone marrow damage.

These five endpoints are distinct, but not necessarily unique indicators of genotoxic and/or cytotoxic damage. Each endpoint is induced by both common kinds of damage or induced uniquely by a specific type of damage. Consequently, experimental protocols that analyze, where feasible, a spectrum of cytogenetic endpoints are a much more powerful investigative tool than are protocols that analyze only one endpoint. Studies on benzene-induced bone marrow damage clearly demonstrate the usefulness of integrating several cytogenetic endpoints into one experimental design (61,65).

Male and female DBA/2 mice (10 to 12 months of age), with and without phenobarbital pretreatment, were exposed to 3,000 ppm of benzene for 4 hours and then exposed to BrdUrd for up to 30 hours. Using routine cytogenetic procedures, the investigators evaluated the frequency of CAs and SCEs and the duration of the cell cycle (i.e., AGT analysis) in bone marrow cells (61,65). Exposure to benzene (see Table 5) (a) induced a significant and equal increase in SCEs in male and female mice, a response that was synergistically enhanced in female but not male mice by PB pretreatment; (b) had no effect on CA frequency unless PB pretreatment occurred, in which case male mice exhibited almost twice as many aberrant cells as did female mice; and (c) caused a significant increase in cell cycle duration in male but not female mice, a response that in this case was synergistically enhanced in male but not female mice by pretreatment with PB. These results indicate the independence of different cytogenetic endpoints and the probability that different metabolites (involving or not involving the parent compound) of benzene are responsible for the different types of bone marrow damage (61,65).

The observation that various cytogenetic indicators of damage are induced independently and involve different metabolites cannot be expected to be unique to benzene. Many chemicals likely induce genotoxic and/or cytotoxic damage through a variety of mechanisms, all of which may not necessarily be induced by the same chemical species/metabolite. It is not possible, based on the above mentioned study, to speculate as to the exact molecular nature of the damaging insult or to which metabolites of benzene are involved. However, these results do demonstrate the

TABLE 5. *Cytogenetic manifestations of genotoxic/cytotoxic damage induced in mouse (DBA/2) bone marrow by a 4-hr exposure to benzene at 3,000 ppm*

Exposure group	Gender[a]	SCE frequency[b]	% Damaged cells[c]	AGT[d] (hr)
Control	Male	4.6 ± 0.2 (6)	8.8 ± 1.2 (5)	14.2 ± 1.3 (6)
	Female	4.5 ± 0.3 (6)	10.8 ± 2.2 (5)	13.4 ± 0.9 (6)
Benzene	Male	8.7 ± 0.4 (10)[e]	12.8 ± 2.0 (5)	16.6 ± 0.4 (7)[e]
	Female	8.2 ± 0.7 (10)[e]	12.0 ± 1.3 (5)	12.2 ± 0.9 (11)
Phenobarbital[f]	Male	4.1 ± 0.2 (7)	10.8 ± 2.0 (5)	11.8 ± 0.4 (7)
	Female	4.2 ± 0.2 (6)	9.6 ± 1.2 (5)	12.5 ± 0.2 (6)
Phenobarbital[f] + benzene	Male	8.3 ± 0.4 (6)[e]	42.4 ± 3.6 (5)[e]	20.9 ± 2.2 (11)[e]
	Female	12.7 ± 1.0 (7)[e]	25.6 ± 1.7 (5)[e]	12.1 ± 0.4 (7)

[a]Ten-month-old mice were exposed to benzene (3,000 ppm; 4 hr) and within the next hour placed on an infusion apparatus and infused i.v. with 50 mg/kg/hr BrdUrd in phosphate buffered saline. The infusion periods ranged from 10 to 30 hr, the animals were injected i.v. with demecolcine (Colcemid) 2 hr before termination. (See ref. 61 for additional details.)
[b]Mean frequency of SCE/cell among animals ± SEM between (n) animals; 25 second-generation metaphase cells were analyzed in each animal.
[c]Mean % damaged cells among animals ± SEM between (n) animals; values reflect the presence of both achromatic lesion, breaks, and rearrangements; 50 first-generation metaphase cells were analyzed in each animal.
[d]Average generation time, mean cell cycle duration ± SEM between (n) animals. See text for method of calculation.
[e]Statistically significant from the appropriate control by Student's t-test at $p < .05$.
[f]Animals were injected intraperitoneally with sodium phenobarbital (50 mg/kg), twice daily for 3 days prior to benzene exposure.

utility of an integrated cytogenetic approach to evaluating bone marrow damage and suggest experiments to evaluate cause-effect relationships.

SUMMARY

Cytogenetic analysis of cytotoxic and/or genotoxic damage in bone marrow is a powerful investigative tool for assessing bone marrow function. Chromosomal aberrations are induced by DNA damage and by alterations in DNA replication. SCEs are also induced by DNA damage, but with different specificity. Micronuclei are induced by both DNA damage and effects on cytokinesis. Aneuploidy is also induced by effects on cytokinesis. Inhibition of cell cycle kinetics is induced by DNA damage and/or nongenotoxic mechanisms. Consequently, the simultaneous assessment of several cytogenetic endpoints permits not only an increased sensitivity but also provides tools for elucidating cause-effect relationships.

ACKNOWLEDGMENTS

Work supported by the U.S. Department of Energy under contract DE-AC02-76CH00016 and for the National Toxicology Program under NIEHS Interagency Agreement YO1-CP-10207, accordingly, the U.S. Government retains a nonexclusive, royalty-free license to publish or reproduce the published form of this contribution, or allow others to do so, for U.S. Government purposes.

REFERENCES

1. Abe, S., and Sasaki, M. (1982): SCE as an index of mutagenesis and/or carcinogenesis. In: *Sister Chromatid Exchange*, edited by A. A. Sandberg, pp. 461–514. Alan R. Liss, New York.
2. Allen, J. W., Shuler, C. F., and Latt, S. A. (1978): Bromodeoxyuridine tablet methodology for *in vivo* studies of DNA synthesis. *Somatic Cell Genet.*, 4:393–405.
3. Barrett, J. F., Wong, A., and McLachlan, J. A. (1981): Diethylstilbestrol induces neoplastic transformation without measurable gene mutation at two loci. *Science*, 212:1402–1404.
4. Bender, M. A. (1980): Relationship of DNA lesions and their repair to chromosomal aberration production. In: *DNA Repair and Mutagenesis in Eukaryotes*, edited by W. M. Generoso, M. D. Shelby, and F. J. deSerres, pp. 245–265. Plenum Press, New York.
5. Bender, M. A., Griggs, H. G., and Bedford, J. (1974): Mechanisms of chromosomal aberration production. III. Chemicals and ionizing radiation. *Mutat. Res.*, 23:197–212.
6. Bessis, M. (1973): *Living Blood Cells and Their Ultrastructure*, translated by R. I. Weed. pp. 191–193. Springer-Verlag, Berlin.
7. Bessis, M. (1973): *Living Blood Cells and Their Ultrastructure*, translated by R. I. Weed, p. 370. Springer-Verlag, Berlin.
8. Bradley, M. O., Hsu, T. C., and Harris, C. C. (1979): Relationship between sister chromatid exchange and mutagenicity, toxicity and DNA damage. *Nature*, 282:318–319.
9. Brenner, S., Pepper, D., Berns, M. W., Tan, E., and Brinkley, B. R. (1981): Kinetochone structure, duplication and distribution in mammalian cells: Analysis by human autoantibodies from scleroderma patients. *J. Cell. Biol.*, 91:95–102.
10. Carrano, A. V., and Thompson, L. H. (1982): Sister chromatid exchange and single-gene mutation. In: *Sister Chromatid Exchange*, edited by S. Wolff, pp. 59–86. John Wiley & Sons, New York.
11. Carrano, A. V., and Wolff, S. (1975): Distribution of sister chromatid exchanges in the euchromatin and heterochromatin of the Indian mutjac. *Chromosoma*, 53:361–369.
12. Cleaver, J. E. (1967): *Thymidine Metabolism and Cell Kinetics*, Elsevier/North Holland, Amsterdam.

13. Chrisman, C. L., and Hinkle, L. L. (1974): Induction of aneuploidy in mouse bone marrow cells with diethylstilbestrol-diphosphate. *Can. J. Genet. Cytol.*, 16:831–835.
14. Darzynkiewicz, Z., Traganos, F., and Melamed, M. R. (1983): Distinction between 5-bromodeoxyuridine labeled and unlabeled mitotic cells by flow cytometry. *Cytometry*, 8:345–348.
15. Evans, H. J. (1974): Effects of ionizing radiation on mammalian chromosomes. In: *Chromosomes and Cancer*, edited by J. German, pp. 191–237. John Wiley & Sons, New York.
16. Evans, H. J., and Scott, D. (1969): The induction of chromosome aberrations by nitrogen mustard and its dependence on DNA synthesis. *Proc. R. Soc. Lond. [Biol.]*, 173:491–512.
17. Gaudin, D. (1973): Some thoughts on a possible relationship between known gene dosage effects and neoplastic transformation. *Theor. Biol.*, 41:191–200.
18. Gray, J. W., Dean, P. N., and Mendelsohn, M. L. (1979): Quantitative cell-cycle analysis. In: *Flow Cytometry and Sorting*, edited by M. R. Melamed, P. F. Mullaney, and M. L. Mendelsohn, pp. 383–407, John Wiley & Sons, New York.
19. Guglielmi, G. E., Vogt, T. F., and Tice, R. R. (1982): Induction of sister chromatid exchanges and inhibition of cellular proliferation *in vitro*. I. Caffeine. *Environ. Mutagen.*, 4:191–200.
20. Heddle, J. A., Hite, M., Kirkhart, B., Mavrournin, K., MacGregor, J. T., Newell, G. W., and Salamone, M. F. (1983): The induction of micronuclei as a measure of genotoxicity. A report of the U.S. Environmental Protection Agency Gene-Tox Program. *Mutat. Res.*, 123:61–118.
21. Ivett, J. L., Luke, C. A., and Tice, R. R. (1984): Range finding studies for determining the optimal doses and termination times for evaluating chromosomal aberrations and sister chromatid exchanges *in vivo*. Presented at the 15th Annual Meeting of the Environmental Mutagen Society. February 19–23, Montreal, Canada, abstract Ha-7.
22. Ivett, J. L., and Tice, R. R. (1981): Diethylstilbestrol-diphosphate induces chromosomal aberrations but not sister chromatid exchanges in murine bone marrow cells *in vivo*. *Environ. Mutagen.*, 3:445–452.
23. Ivett, J. L., and Tice, R. R. (1984): Average generation time: A new method for analyzing cellular proliferation kinetics based on bromodeoxyuridine-dependent chromosomal differential staining patterns. *Environ. Mutagen.* (submitted).
24. King, M.-T., Wild, D., Gocke, E., and Eckhardt, K. (1982): 5-Bromodeoxyuridine tablets with improved depot effect for analysis *in vivo* of sister chromatid exchanges in bone marrow and spermatogonial cells. *Mutat. Res.*, 97:117–129.
25. Laerum, O. D., Lindmo, T., and Thorud, E., editors (1981): Flow cytometry. IV. Proceedings of the IVth International Symposium in Flow Cytometry (Pulse Cytophotometry). Acta Path. *Microbiologica*, Section A.
26. Latt, S. A. (1973): Microfluorometric detection of deoxyribounucleic acid replication in human metaphase chromosomes. *Proc. Natl. Acad. Sci. USA*, 70:3395–3399.
27. Latt, S. A., Allen, J. W., Rogers, W. E., and Juergens, L. A. (1977): *In vitro* and *in vivo* analysis of sister chromatid exchange formation. In: *Handbook of Mutagenicity Test Procedures*, edited by B. J. Kilbey, M. Legator, W. Nichols, and C. Ramel, pp. 275–291. Elsevier Scientific Publishing Co., New York.
28. Liang, J. C., and Hsu, T. C. (1984): Induction of aneuploidy by mitotic arrestants in mammalian cell cultures. Presented at the 15th Annual Meeting of the Environmental Mutagen Society, February 19–23, Montreal, Canada, abstract Fa-2.
29. Littlefield, L. G. (1982): Effects of DNA-damaging agents on SCE. In: *Sister Chromatid Exchange*, edited by A. A. Sandberg, pp. 355–394. Alan R. Liss, New York.
30. Luke, C. A., Tice, R. R., Sawey, M. J., Ormiston, B. G., and Bosler, E. M. (1984): Environmental biomonitoring: The feasibility of using feral mouse populations to detect genotoxic pollutants. Presented at the 15th Annual Meeting of the Environmental Mutagen Society, February 19-23, Montreal, Canada, abstract cb-7.
31. MagGregor, J. T., Wehr, C. M., and Gould, D. H. (1980): Clastogen-induced micronuclei in peripheral blood erythrocytes: The basis of an improved micronucleus test. *Environ. Mutagen.*, 2:509–514.
32. McFee, A. F., Lowe, K. W., San Sebastion, J. R. (1983): Improved sister chromatid differentiation using paraffin-coated bromodeoxyuridine tablets in mice. *Mutat. Res.*, 119:83–88.
33. McFee, A. F., Lowe, K. W., and Sherrill, M. N. (1983): Influence of time on the *in vivo* induction of sister chromatid exchanges and chromosomal aberrations. Presented at the 15th Annual Meeting of the Environmental Mutagen Society, February 19-23, Montreal, Canada, abstract Ha-10.
34. McFee, A. F., and Tice, R. R. (1984): (Unpublished data).

35. Miller, V. M., and Tice, R. R. (1984): The induction of micronuclei in peripheral blood erythrocytes by ionizing radiation: Kinetics of expression and residual damage. Presented at the 15th Annual Meeting of the Environmental Mutagen Society, February 19-23, Montreal, Canada, abstract Cb-7.
36. Mitelman, F. (1983): Chromosome patterns in human cancer and leukemia. In: *Chromosomes and Cancer, from Molecules to Man*, edited by J. D. Rowley and J. E. Ultmann, Bristol-Myers Cancer Symposium, Vol. 5. pp. 61–84. Academic Press, Orlando.
37. Morimoto, K., Sato, M., and Koizumi, A. (1983): Proliferative kinetics of human lymphocytes in culture measured by autoradiography and sister chromatid differential staining. *Exp. Cell Res.*, 145:345–356.
38. Morris, S. M., Beranek, D. J., and Heflich, R. H. (1983): The relationship between sister chromatid exchange induction and the formation of specific methylated DNA adducts in CHO cells. *Mutat. Res.*, 121:261.
39. Ormiston, B. G., Luke, C. A., and Tice, R. R. (1985): The Syrian golden hamster: Another species for the peripheral blood micronucleus assay. *Mutat. Res. (submitted)*.
40. Pedersen-Bjergaard, J., Vindelov, L., Philip, P., Ruutu, P., Elmgreen, J., Repo, H., Christensen, I. J., Killmann, S. A., and Jensen, G. (1983): Acute nonlymphocytic leukemia, preleukemia and acute myeloproliferative syndrome secondary to treatment of other malignant diseases. Clinical and cytogenetic characteristics and results on *in vitro* culture of bone marrow and HLA typing. *Blood*, 60:172–179.
41. Perry, P., and Evans, H. J. (1975): Cytological detetion of mutagen-carcinogen exposure by sister chromatid exchange. *Nature*, 258:121–124.
42. Preston, R. J., Au, W., Bender, M. A., Brewen, J. G., Carrano, A. V., Heddle, J. A., McFee, A. F., Wolff, S., and Wassom, J. S. (1983): Mammalian *in vivo* and *in vitro* cytogenetic assays: A report of the Gene-Tox Program. *Mutat. Res.*, 87:143–188.
43. Reynolds, R. J., Natarajan, A. T., and Lohman, P. H. M. (1979): *Micrococcus luteus* endonuclease-sensitive sites and sister chromatid exchanges in Chinese hamster ovary cells. *Mutat. Res.*, 64:353–356.
44. Sandberg, A. A. (1982): *Sister Chromatid Exchange*, Program and Topics in Cytogenetics, Vol. 2. Alan R. Liss, New York.
45. Sasaki, M. (1982): Sister chromatid exchange as a reflection of cellular DNA repair. In: *Sister Chromatid Exchange*, edited by A. A. Sandberg, pp. 135–164, Alan R. Liss, New York.
46. Satya-Prakash, K. L., and Liang, J. C. (1984): Induction of aneupolidy and chromosome breakage by mitotic arrestants, vinblastine and colcemid in mouse bone marrow. Presented at the 15th Annual Meeting of the Environmental Mutagen Society. February 19–23, Montreal, Canada, abstract Fa-3.
47. Savage, J. R. K. (1975): Classification and relationships of induced chromosomal structural changes. *J. Med. Genet.*, 12:103–122.
48. Sawada, M., and Ishidate, Jr, M. (1978): Colchicine-like effect of diethylstibestrol (DES) on mammalian cells *in vitro*. *Mutat. Res.*, 57:175–182.
49. Schlegel, R., and MacGregor, J. T. (1982): The persistance of micronuclei in peripheral blood erythrocytes: Detection of chronic chromosome breakage in mice. *Mutat. Res.*, 104:367–369.
50. Schlegel, R., and MacGregor, J. T. (1984): The persistance of micronucleated erythrocytes in the peripheral circulation of normal and splenectomized Fisher 344 rats: Implications for cytogenetic screening. *Mutat. Res.*, *(in press)*.
51. Schmid, W. (1976): The micronucleus test for cytogenetic analysis. In: *Chemical Mutagen*, Vol. 4, edited by A. Hollaender, pp. 31–53. Plenum Press, New York.
52. Schneider, E. L., Nakanishi, Y., Lewis, J., and Sternberg, H. (1981): Simultaneous examination of sister chromatid exchanges and cell replication kinetics in tumor and normal cells *in vivo*. *Cancer Res.*, 41:4973–4975.
53. Schneider, E. L., Sternberg, H., and Tice, R. R. (1977): *In vivo* analysis of cellular replication. *Proc. Natl. Acad. Sci. USA*, 74:2041–2044.
54. Schneider, E. L., Tice, R. R., and Kram, D. (1978): Bromodeoxyuridine differential chromatid staining technique: A new approach to examining sister chromatid exchange and cell replication kinetics. In: *Methods in Cell Biology*, Vol. II, edited by D. M. Prescott, pp. 379–409. Academic Press, New York.
55. Schubert, I., and Rieger, R. (1981): Sister chromatid exchanges and heterochromatin. *Hum. Genet.*, 57:119–130.

56. Schvartzman, J. B., and Tice, R. R. (1982): 5-Bromodeoxyuridine and its role in the production of sister chromatid exchange. In: *Sister Chromatid Exchange*, edited by A. A. Sandberg, pp. 123–134. Alan R. Liss, New York.

57. Shafer, D. A. (1982): Alternative replication bypass mechanisms for sister chromatid exchange formation. In: *Sister Chromatid Exchange*, edited by A. A. Sandberg, pp. 67–98. Alan R. Liss, New York.

58. Takehisa, S. (1982): Induction of sister chromatid exchanges by chemical agents. In: *Sister Chromatid Exchange*, edited by S. Wolff, pp. 87–148, John Wiley and Sons, New York.

59. Taylor, J. H. (1958): Sister chromatid exchanges in tritium labeled chromosomes. *Genetics*, 43:515–529.

60. Tice, R. R., Chaillet, J., and Schneider, E. L. (1975): Evidence derived from sister chromatid exchanges of restricted rejoining of chromatid subunits. *Nature*, 256:642–643.

61. Tice, R. R., Costa, D. L., and Drew, R. T. (1980): Cytogenetic effects of inhaled benzene in murine bone marrow: Induction of sister chromatid exchanges, chromosomal aberrations, and cellular proliferation inhibition in DBA/2 mice. *Proc. Natl. Acad. Sci. USA*, 77:2148–2152.

62. Tice, R. R., Luke, C., Miller, V., McFee, A. F., and San Sebastion, J. (1983): The *in vivo* mouse bone marrow cytogenetic bioassay. 1. Evaluation of acute exposure protocols and sister chromatid exchange (SCE) response. Presented at the 14th Annual Meeting of the Environmental Mutagen Society, March 3-6, San Antonio, TX, abstract Bb-6.

63. Tice, R. R., Sawey, J. J., Drew, R. T., and Cronkite, E. P. (1984): Benzene-induced micronuclei in the peripheral blood of mice: A retrospective analysis. Presented at the 15th Annual Meeting of the Environmental Mutagen Society, February 19-23, Montreal, Canada, abstract Fa-1.

64. Tice, R. R., and Schvartzman, J. B. (1982): Sister chromatid exchange: A measure of DNA lesion persistance. In: *Sister Chromatid Exchange*, edited by A. A. Sandberg, pp. 33–46. Alan R. Liss, New York.

65. Tice, R. R., Vogt, T. F., and Costa, D. L. (1982): Cytogenetic effects of inhaled benzene in murine bone marrow. In: *Genotoxic Effects of Airborne Agents*, edited by R. R. Tice, D. L. Costa, and K. M. Schaich, pp. 257–275. Plenum Press, New York.

66. Vaughan-Dellarco, V. L., Marvournin, K. H., and Tice, R. R. (1985): Aneuploidy and health risk assessment: Future directions. *Environ. Mutagen. (submitted)*.

67. Whorton, E. B., Jr. (1983): Statistical design, analysis, and interference issues in studies using SCE. In: *Sister Chromatid Exchange: Twenty-Five Years of Experimental Research, Book A: The Nature of SCE*, edited by R. R. Tice, and A. Hollaendar, Plenum Press, New York. pp. 431–440.

68. Whorton, E. B., Jr., Bee, D. E., and Kilian, D. J. (1979): Variations in the proportion of abnormal cells and required sample sizes for human cytogenetic studies. *Mutat. Res.*, 64:79–86.

69. Wolff, S. (1982): Chromosome aberrations, sister chromatid exchanges, and the lesions that produce them. In: *Sister Chromatid Exchange*, edited by S. Wolff, pp. 41–58. John Wiley & Sons, New York.

70. Wolff, S., editor (1982): *Sister Chromatid Exchange*, John Wiley & Sons, New York.

71. Wolff, S., Bodycote, J., and Painter, R. B. (1974): Sister chromatid exchanges induced in Chinese hamster cells by UV irradiation at different stages of the cell cycle: The necessity of cells to pass through S. *Mutat. Res.*, 25:73–81.

72. Yamamoto, K. I., and Kikuchi, Y. (1980): A comparison of diameters of micronuclei induced by clastogens and by spindle poisons. *Mutat. Res.*, 71:127–131.

Toxicology of the Blood and Bone Marrow,
edited by Richard D. Irons. Raven Press,
New York © 1985.

Metabolism of Benzene and Its Metabolites in Bone Marrow

*Tadashi Sawahata,[1] *Douglas E. Rickert, and
†William F. Greenlee

*Departments of *General and Biochemical Toxicology and †Cell Biology, Chemical
Industry Institute of Toxicology, Research Triangle Park, North Carolina 27709*

Chronic exposure to benzene (25 to 1,000 ppm) is characterized by a progressive degeneration of bone marrow and dysfunction of the hemopoietic system. In the peripheral blood, lymphocytopenia is one of the most sensitive and easily measured indicators of benzene toxicity. Extensive studies during the past decade have provided considerable evidence that the expression of benzene toxicity requires metabolism of the parent compound to one or more toxic species (for reviews see refs. 19 and 34). This chapter reviews the available information on the metabolism of benzene and its primary metabolites, phenol, catechol, and hydroquinone in the bone marrow and details putative reaction pathways for the formation of covalent adducts.

METABOLISM OF BENZENE IN THE LIVER

In the liver benzene is metabolized to phenol (via benzene oxide) by the cytochrome P-450 monooxygenase system (Fig. 1) (9). The majority of benzene oxide formed spontaneously rearranges to yield phenol (37), with a small portion of the oxide undergoing hydrolysis (catalyzed by epoxide hydrolase) to benzene-1,2-trans-dihydrodiol. The dihydrodiol can be further converted to catechol by cytosolic dehydrogenase (17). This is believed to be the major metabolic pathway from benzene to catechol (27,35).

Phenol can be further hydroxylated by the cytochrome P-450-dependent monooxygenase system to hydroquinone and catechol, the former being the major product (30,38). Different isozymes of cytochrome P-450 may be involved in the formation of hydroquinone and catechol (30). Hydroquinone and catechol are believed to be the immediate precursors of the ultimate reactive metabolites responsible for the covalent binding seen during the metabolism of benzene by hepatic microsomes (30,38). By analogy with catecholamines and catechol estrogens (5,20,22,31), the

---

[1]*Present address:* Toxicology Laboratory, Toray Industries, Inc., 2-7-35 Sonoyama, Otsu 520, Japan.

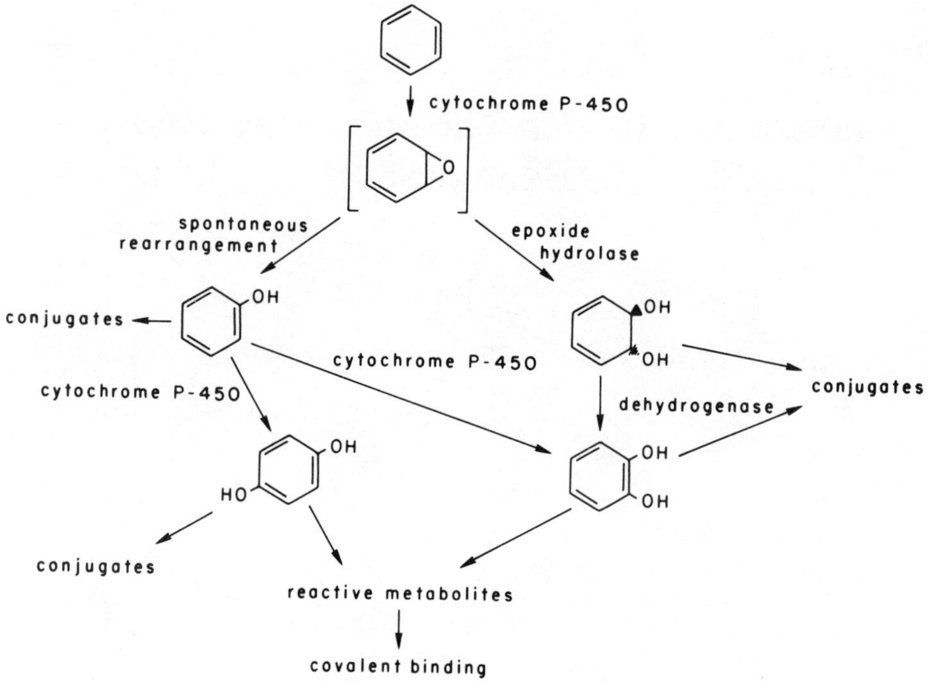

FIG. 1.   Pathways for benzene metabolism in liver.

ultimate reactive forms of the dihydroxy metabolites of benzene are postulated to be semiquinone radicals and/or benzoquinones (38). Tunek et al. (39) reported that a single microsomal protein (MW 72,000) is selectively radiolabeled when radioactive benzene or phenol is incubated with microsomes in the presence of reduced nicotinamide adenine dinucleotide phosphate (NADPH). Such selective covalent binding suggests that this protein, which does not appear to be cytochrome P-450 (MW 48,000 to 54,000) (12), participates in the formation of the ultimate reactive metabolites. The identity and enzymatic properties of this protein are not known.

METABOLISM OF BENZENE IN BONE MARROW

Andrews et al. (1) reported that benzene metabolites accumulate in the bone marrow when benzene is administered to mice subcutaneously. The major metabolites detected were the glucuronide and ethereal sulfate conjugates of phenol. Free phenol and the glucuronide and ethereal sulfate conjugates of catechol were also present but accounted for only 10% of the metabolites. Administration of radiolabeled phenol, phenyl glucuronide, or phenyl sulfate did not result in accumulation of radioactivity in the bone marrow, and the authors suggested that the high concentrations of benzene metabolites in the bone marrow following benzene administration were due to benzene metabolism by that tissue.

The concentration of cytochrome P-450 measured in bone marrow is low ($<5\%$) compared with that measured in liver or lung (2,40) (Table 1). The metabolism of benzene by rabbit bone marrow microsomes requires NADPH and is inhibited by carbon monoxide. Phenol and an unidentified metabolite were formed at rates of 89 and 25 pmole/mg protein/45 min, respectively, when benzene was incubated with rabbit bone marrow microsomes in the presence of an NADPH-generating system (2), but the total amount of phenol formed was less than 0.24% of the benzene added. Perfusion of an isolated rat femur with blood containing [^{14}C]benzene at a concentration 200- to 800-fold greater than the reported concentrations of toxic doses of benzene to mice or rats (2,25) resulted in the formation of free phenol, catechol, hydroquinone, and an unidentified compound (15). The total metabolites recovered from blood and bone marrow accounted for only $2 \times 10^{-4}\%$ of the administered dose. The results of these studies suggest that the metabolism of benzene by bone marrow cannot account for the concentration of metabolites reported in that tissue *in vivo* (1,25).

Phenol, hydroquinone, and catechol are more toxic to bone marrow cultures than benzene (13), and they are mitotic inhibitors (23). The accumulation of these phenolic metabolites of benzene in the bone marrow has been studied in rats exposed to benzene (500 ppm) for 6 hours by inhalation. Free phenol, hydroquinone, and catechol were detected not only in blood, but also in bone marrow (25). Phenol concentrations in both blood and bone marrow rapidly decreased after the exposure was terminated. In contrast, the concentrations of hydroquinone and catechol in bone marrow and blood remained essentially unchanged for at least 9 hours after exposure to benzene stopped. Studies on the disposition of ^{14}C-labeled benzene metabolites using whole-body autoradiography indicated that radioactivity associated with hydroquinone or catechol, but not phenol, concentrated in the bone marrow and lymphoid organs (10). The amounts of radioactivity associated with hydroquinone and catechol in these tissues were reduced in rats pretreated with Arochlor 1254, a regimen that protects against benzene toxicity (10).

The relative contribution of hepatic and bone marrow cell metabolism of benzene in the expression of toxicity is poorly understood at present. However, the available

TABLE 1. *Concentration of the cytochrome P-450-containing monooxygenase system in the liver, lung, and bone marrow*

Tissue	Cytochrome P-450[a]	NADPH-cytochrome c reductase[b]
Liver[c]	810–1,700	90–238
Lung[c]	270–380	58–94
Bone marrow[d] (rabbit)	26–51	7.8–21

[a]pmole/mg microsomal protein.
[b]pmoles of cytochrome c reduced/mg microsomal protein/min.
[c]Data from (40).
[d]Data from (2).

data suggest that the retention of hydroquinone and catechol in bone marrow of rats exposed to benzene by inhalation (25) could result from the formation of these compounds in the liver and subsequent uptake by bone marrow cells. The importance of hepatic metabolism of benzene in production of hydroxy metabolites found in the bone marrow is supported by the experiments performed by Sammett et al. (26). They found that partial hepatectomy resulted not only in a reduction in amounts of benzene metabolites excreted in urine, but also in a decrease in concentrations of benzene metabolites detected in bone marrow.

METABOLISM AND COVALENT BINDING OF HYDROXYLATED BENZENE METABOLITES IN BONE MARROW

Tunek et al. (37) suggested that covalently bound metabolites of benzene formed during incubations of benzene with rat liver microsomes resulted from further metabolism of phenol rather than from the reaction of benzene oxide with macromolecules. *In vivo* studies have indicated that phenol and other hydroxylated metabolites of benzene are present in bone marrow after benzene administration. Bone marrow contains relatively low concentrations of cytochrome P-450-dependent monooxygenases (Table 1); thus, the metabolism of hydroxylated benzene metabolites in bone marrow by enzyme systems other than the cytochrome P-450-dependent monooxygenases has been investigated. Peroxidases are present in the bone marrow (4,14) and are capable of oxidation of phenols (3). The oxidation of phenol by horseradish peroxidase (HRP) has been used as an *in vitro* model for the bone marrow peroxidases. Danner et al. (3) reported that the oxidation of phenol by HRP in the presence of hydrogen peroxide resulted in the formation of *o,o'*-biphenol as the only metabolite. In contrast, Sawahata and Neal (29) reported that HRP catalyzed the conversion of phenol to *o,o'*-biphenol, *p,p'*-biphenol, and *p*-diphenoquinone. The biphenols were also formed during hydrogen peroxide-dependent metabolism of phenol by a homogenate of red blood cell-free bone marrow cells (29). No formation of *p*-diphenoquinone was observed but covalent binding of phenol-related material to protein was extensive. Covalently bound materal accounted for more than 90% of the phenol metabolized (Sawahata and Neal, *unpublished observations*). Both the formation of biphenols and the covalent binding of phenol to protein were inhibited by the potent peroxidase inhibitors cyanide and azide.

A partially purified myeloperoxidase preparation from rat bone marrow also catalyzed the oxidation of phenol in the presence of hydrogen peroxide. *p*-Diphenoquinone accounted for 95% of the metabolites formed; lesser amounts of *o,o'*- and *p,p'*-biphenols were formed (Sawahata and Neal, *unpublished observations*). Inclusion of bovine serum albumin in the incubation mixtures resulted in a decrease in the formation of *p*-diphenoquinone accompanied by an increase in the levels of covalent binding of metabolites to protein. This is the first demonstration that a mammalian peroxidase can catalyze activation of a phenol and suggests that *p*-diphenoquinone is the active metabolite (Fig. 2).

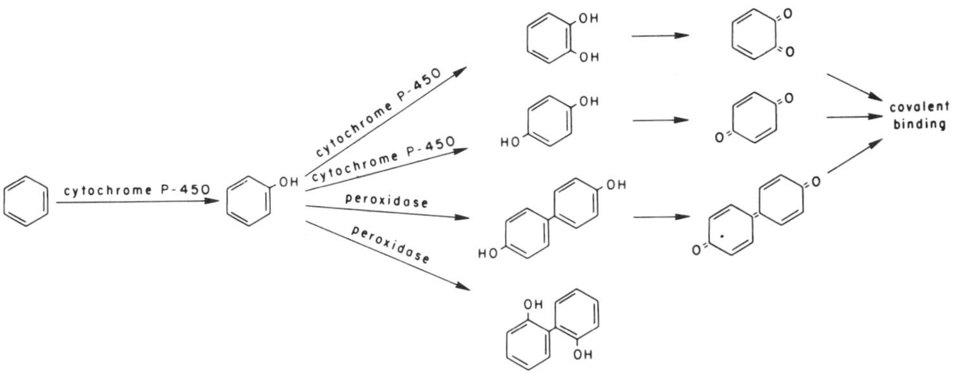

FIG. 2. Postulated pathways for benzene metabolism in bone marrow. Conversion of the alcohols to the quinones can occur by autooxidation and may also occur via the actions of peroxidases (see text).

Reactive metabolites of benzene covalently bind to macromolecules in bone marrow after administration to mice (33), or during metabolism of benzene by isolated perfused rat femur (15). The latter findings indicate that bone marrow can generate reactive metabolites from benzene, although the contribution of bone marrow to total benzene metabolism *in vivo* is likely to be small (see above). Concentrations of covalently bound material due to benzene administration were reduced in animals pretreated with Arochlor 1254 (11). Pretreatment with Arochlor 1254 also protected animals from benzene-induced lymphocytopenia (10). Partial hepatectomy alleviated benzene-induced depression of erythropoiesis and decreased the concentrations of covalently bound benzene metabolites to macromolecules in bone marrow (26). Thus, manipulations that alter the covalent binding of benzene to bone marrow macromolecules also alter some manifestations of its toxicity to bone marrow.

Gill and Ahmed (7) reported that covalent binding of benzene in bone marrow is predominantly to DNA rather than to protein and that in the liver, macromolecules of the mitochondrial fractions are most extensively labeled after radiolabeled benzene administration. Kalf et al. (18) reported that benzene metabolites bind to mitochondrial DNA when benzene is incubated with bone marrow mitoplasts in the presence of NADPH. Incubation of benzene with bone marrow mitoplasts also results in an inhibition of mitochondrial RNA synthesis. It was hypothesized that the covalent binding of benzene metabolites to mitochondrial DNA inhibits transcription by mitochondrial RNA polymerase.

Mitochondrial cytochrome P-450 was suggested to be involved in the formation of reactive metabolites responsible for covalent binding to mitochondrial DNA (7), but whether reactive metabolites are formed directly from benzene or from its metabolites is uncertain. If the reactive metabolite(s) is formed from benzene, it is possible that bone marrow mitochondrial cytochrome P-450 converts benzene to benzene oxide, which covalently binds to mitochondrial DNA. Unidentified metabolites were detected in bone marrow microsomal incubations containing benzene (2) as well as in bone marrow perfusion experiments (15), but it is not known whether the unidentified metabolites were the same in both systems, whether they represented further metabolic products of phenol, catechol, or hydroquinone, or whether they were precursors to the metabolites that covalently bound to bone marrow macromolecules.

The administration of radioactive hydroquinone or catechol results in significant covalent binding of radioactivity to bone marrow macromolecules (11). The reactive metabolites derived from hydroquinone and catechol are likely to be semiquinones and/or quinones. Benzoquinone is a more potent suppressor of mitogen response and inhibitor for tubulin polymerization than hydroquinone (16). Catechol exhibits no effect on microtubule assembly but completely inhibits tubulin polymerization in the presence of tyrosinase (16), which catalyzes the oxidation of catechol directly to o-benzoquinone without releasing semiquinone radical intermediates (21). Benzoquinones readily react with sulfhydryl-containing amino acids (30), and their suppressive effects on mitogen response may be due to modification of sulfhydryl groups (16). This is supported by experiments with sulfhydryl reagents such as N-ethylmaleimide and cytochalasin A (6,8,36), which produce similar effects.

There are several pathways for the conversion of the hydroxylated metabolites of benzene to semiquinones or quinones. Both hydroquinone and 1,2,4-benzenetriol autooxidize at physiologic pH in the presence of oxygen (11). The ultraviolet absorption spectrum of the autooxidation product of hydroquinone is identical to that of benzoquinone. Superoxide anion radical (as determined indirectly by adrenochrome formation from epinephrine) is generated during the autooxidation of hydroquinone and 1,2,4-benzenetriol (11). Thus, it is possible that in the bone marrow both hydroquinone and 1,2,4-benzenetriol form semiquinones, quinones, and the potentially toxic superoxide anion radical. Alternatively, it is possible that myeloperoxidase is involved in the conversion of hydroquinone and catechol to semiquinones or quinones, as bone marrow contains high concentrations of this enzyme (Sawahata and Neal, *unpublished data*) and as both compounds are known to be oxidized to quinones via semiquinone radicals by peroxidases (24,28,42). Myeloperoxidase-mediated oxidation of phenol to p-diphenoquinone may also be of importance in the hematopoietic toxicity of benzene.

Finally, phenols have been shown to react with oxyhemoglobin, resulting in the formation of phenoxy radicals, methemoglobin, and hydrogen peroxide (41):

$$Hb\text{-}O_2 + PhOH \rightarrow metHb + PhO^{\bullet} + H_2O_2$$

The resulting methemoglobin and hydrogen peroxide comprise a peroxidase system that also can catalyze the oxidation of phenol to form phenoxy radicals (32). The methemoglobin-hydrogen peroxide system thus formed may also be of toxicological importance.

It is clear that there are a number of metabolic pathways for benzene that could result in the formation of metabolites capable of interacting with critical bone marrow constituents. Currently, none of the pathways discussed above can be unequivocally dismissed. Much more work is needed to determine which, if any, of the postulated pathways is (are) correct. It is unlikely that such a determination can be made until there is a consensus concerning the events that lead, on a molecular level, to the expression of benzene toxicity.

REFERENCES

1. Andrews, L. S., Lee, E. W., Witmer, C. M., Kocsis, J. J., and Snyder, R. (1977): Effects of toluene on the metabolism, disposition and hemopoietic toxicity of [^{14}C]benzene. *Biochem. Pharmacol.*, 26:293–300.
2. Andrews, L. S., Sasame, H. A., and Gillette, J. R. (1979): ^{3}H-benzene metabolism in rabbit bone marrow. *Life Sci.*, 25:567–572.
3. Danner, D. J., Brignac, D., Jr., Archeneaux, D., and Patel, V. (1973): The oxidation of phenol and its reaction product by horseradish peroxidase and hydrogen peroxide. *Arch. Biochem. Biophys.*, 156:759–763.
4. Desser, R. K., Himmelhoch, S. R., Evans, W. H., Januska, M., Mage, M., and Shelton, E. (1972): Guinea pig heterophil and eosinophil peroxidase. *Arch. Biochem. Biophys.*, 148:452–465.
5. Dybing, E., Nelson, S. D., Mitchell, J. R., Sasame, H. A., and Gillette, J. R. (1976): Oxidation of α-methyldopa and other catechols by cytochrome P-450-generated superoxide anion: Possible mechanism of methyldopa hepatitis. *Mol. Pharmacol.*, 12:911–920.
6. Elferink, J. G. R., and Riemersa, J. C. (1980): Effects of sulfhydryl reagent on phagocytosis and exocytosis in rabbit polymorphonuclear leukocytes. *Chem. Biol. Interact.*, 30:139–149.
7. Gill, D. P., and Ahmed, A. E. (1981): Covalent binding of benzene to cellular organelles and bone marrow nucleic acids. *Biochem. Pharmacol.*, 30:1127–1131.
8. Giordano, G. I., and Lichtman, M. A. (1973): The role of sulfhydryl groups in human neutrophile adhesion, movement and particle ingestion. *J. Cell Physiol.*, 82:387–396.
9. Gonasun, L. M., Witmer, C., Kocsis, J. J., and Snyder, R. (1973): Benzene metabolism in mouse liver microsomes. *Toxicol. Appl. Pharmacol.*, 26:398–406.
10. Greenlee, W. F., Gross, E. A., and Irons, R. D. (1981): Relationship between toxicity and the disposition of ^{14}C-labelled benzene metabolites in the rat. *Chem. Biol. Interact.*, 33:285–299.
11. Greenlee, W. F., Sun, J. D., and Bus, J. S. (1981): A proposed mechanism of benzene toxicity: Formation of reactive intermediates from polyphenol metabolites. *Toxicol. Appl. Pharmacol.*, 59:187–195.
12. Guengerich, F. P. (1977): Separation and purification of multiple forms of microsomal cytochrome P-450: Activity of different forms of cytochrome P-450 towards several compounds of environmental interest. *J. Biol. Chem.*, 252:3970–3979.
13. Harrison, K., and Randoll, F. W. (1948): An application of bone marrow cultures to toxicology and therapeutics. *Q. J. Exp. Physiol.*, 34:141–150.
14. Himmelhoch, S. R., Evans, W. H., Mage, M. G., and Peterson, E. A. (1969): Purification of myeloperoxidase from the bone marrow of the guinea pig. *Biochemistry*, 8:914–921.
15. Irons, R. D., Dent, J. G., Baker, T. S., and Rickert, D. E. (1980): Benzene is metabolized and covalently bound in bone marrow *in situ*. *Chem. Biol. Interact.*, 30:241–245.
16. Irons, R. D., Neptun, D. A., and Pfeifer, R. W. (1981): Inhibition of lymphocyte transformation and microtubule assembly by quinone metabolites of benzene: Evidence for a common mechanism. *J. Reticuloendothel. Soc.*, 30:359–372.
17. Jerina, D., Daly, J., Witkop, B., Zaltzman-Nirenberg, P., and Undenfriend, S. (1968): Role of the arene oxide-oxepin system in the metabolism of aromatic substrates. I. *In Vitro* conversion of benzene oxide to a premercapturic acid and a dihydrodiol. *Arch. Biochem. Biophys.*, 128:176–183.
18. Kalf, G. F., Rushmore, T., and Snyder, R. (1982): Benzene inhibits RNA synthesis in mitochondria from liver and bone marrow. *Chem. Biol. Interact.*, 42:353–370.
19. Laskin, S., and Goldstein, B. D., editors (1977): Benzene toxicity: A critical evaluation. *J. Toxicol. Environ. Health*, [Suppl. 2].
20. Marks, F., and Hechker, E. (1969): Metabolism and mechanism of action of oestrogens. XII. Structure and mechanism of formation of watersoluble and protein bound metabolites of oestrone in rat liver microsomes *in vitro* and *in vivo*. *Biochim. Biophys. Acta*, 187:250–265.
21. Mason, H. S., Spencer, E., and Yamazaki, I. (1961): Identification by electron spin resonance

spectroscopy of the primary product of tyrosinase-catalyzed catechol oxidation. *Biochem. Biophys. Res. Commun.*, 4:236–238.

22. Nelson, S. D., Mitchell, J. R., Dybing, E., and Sasame, H. A. (1976): Cytochrome P-450 mediated oxidation of 2-hydroxylestrogens to reactive intermediates. *Biochem. Biophys. Res. Commun.*, 70:1157–1165.

23. Parmentier, R., and Dustin, P., Jr. (1953): On the mechanism of the mitotic abnormalities induced by hydroquinone in animal tissues. *Rev. Belge. Pathol. Med. Exp.*, 23:20–30.

24. Pugh, C. E. M., and Raper, H. S. (1927): CLXXX. The action of tyrosinase on phenols. With some observations on the classification of oxidases. *Biochem. J.*, 21:1370–1383.

25. Rickert, D. E., Baker, T. S., Bus, J. S., Barrow, C. S., and Irons, R. D. (1979): Benzene disposition in the rat after exposure by inhalation. *Toxicol. Appl. Pharmacol.*, 49:417–423.

26. Sammett, D., Lee, E. W., Kocsis, J. J., and Snyder, R. (1979): Partial hepatectomy reduces both metabolism and toxicity of benzene. *J. Toxicol. Environ. Health*, 5:785–792.

27. Sato, T., Fukuyama, T., Suzuki, T., and Yoshikawa, H. (1963): 1,2,-Dihydro-1,2,-dihydroxybenzene and several other substances in the metabolism of benzene. *J. Biochem. (Tokyo)*, 53:23–27.

28. Sawada, Y., Iyanagi, T., and Yamazaki, I. (1975): Relation between redox potential and rate constants in reaction coupled with system oxygen-superoxide. *Biochemistry*, 14:3761–3764.

29. Sawahata, T., and Neal, R. A. (1982): Horseradish peroxidase-mediated oxidation of phenol. *Biochem. Biophys. Res. Commun.*, 109:988–994.

30. Sawahata, T., and Neal, R. A. (1983): Hydrogen peroxide-dependent metabolism of phenol in bone marrow. Myeloperoxidase-mediated oxidation of phenol. *Mol. Pharmacol.*, 23:453–460.

31. Scheulen, M., Wollenberg, P., Bolt, H. M., Kappus, H., and Remmer, H. (1975): Irreversible binding of dopa and dopamine metabolites to protein by rat liver microsomes. *Biochem. Biophys. Res. Commun.*, 66:1396–1400.

32. Shiga, T., and Imaizumi, K. (1973): Generation of phenoxy radicals by methemoglobin-hydrogen peroxide studied by electron paramagnetic resonance. *Arch. Biochem. Biophys.*, 154:540–547.

33. Snyder, R., Lee, E. W., and Kocsis, J. J. (1978): Binding of labeled benzene metabolites to mouse liver and bone marrow. *Res. Commun. Chem. Path. Pharmacol.*, 20:191–194.

34. Snyder, R., Longacre, S. L., Witmer, C. M., Kocsis, J. J., Andrews, L. A., and Lee, E. W. (1981): Biochemical toxicology of benzene. In: *Reviews in Biochemical Toxicology*, edited by E. Hodgson, J. R. Bend, and R. M. Philpot, Vol. 3, pp. 123–153. Elsevier/North-Holland, New York.

35. Tomaszewski, J. E., Jerina, D. M., and Daly, J. W. (1975): Deuterium isotope effects during formation of phenols by hepatic monooxygenases. Evidence for an alternative to the arene oxide pathway. *Biochemistry*, 14:2024–2031.

36. Tsan, M., Newman, B., and McIntyre, P. A. (1976): Surface sulfhydryl groups and phagocytosis-associated oxidative metabolic changes in human polymorphonuclear leucocytes. *Br. J. Hemat.*, 33:189–204.

37. Tunek, A., Platt, K. L., Bentley, P., and Oesch, F. (1978): Microsomal metabolism of benzene to species irreversibly binding to microsomal protein and effects of modifications of this metabolism. *Mol. Pharmacol.*, 14:920–929.

38. Tunek, A., Platt, K. L., Pryzybylski, M., and Oesch, F. (1980): Multi-step metabolic activation of benzene. Effect of superoxide dismutase on covalent binding to microsomal macromolecules, and identification of glutathione conjugates using high pressure liquid chromatography and field desorption mass spectrometry. *Chem. Biol. Interact.*, 33:1–17.

39. Tunek, A., Schelin, C., and Jergil, B. (1979): Microsomal target proteins of metabolically activated aromatic hydrocarbons. *Chem. Biol. Interact.*, 27:133–144.

40. Vainio, H., and Hietanen, E. (1980): Role of extrahepatic metabolism. In: *Concepts in Drug Metabolism*, edited by P. Jenner and B. Testa, Part A, pp. 251–284, Marcel Dekker, New York.

41. Wallence, W. J., and Caughey, W. S. (1975): Mechanism for the autoxidation of hemoglobin by phenols, nitrite and "oxidant" drugs. Peroxide formation by one electron donation to bound dioxygen. *Biochem. Biophys. Res. Commun.*, 62:561–567.

42. Yamazaki, I., Mason, H. S., and Piette, L. (1960): Identification, by electron paramagnetic resonance spectroscopy, of free radicals generated from substrates by peroxidase. *J. Biol. Chem.*, 235:2444–2449.

Toxicology of the Blood and Bone Marrow,
edited by Richard D. Irons. Raven Press,
New York © 1985.

Occupational Factors in the Epidemiology of Chemically Induced Lymphoid and Hemopoietic Cancers

Theodora A. Tsongas[1]

Office of Standards Review, Health Standards Program, Occupational Safety and Health Administration, U.S. Department of Labor, Washington, D.C. 20210

This chapter reviews the available epidemiologic literature on malignant proliferative disorders of the lymphoid and hemopoietic systems (leukemia, lymphoma,
and multiple myeloma) for which there is evidence of an association with employment in certain occupations. The purpose of this review is to examine the evidence
on chemical induction of these cancers in humans and to identify common etiologic
features of these cancers if they are discernible from human data. An essential
part of this review is the discussion of difficulties that may arise in the collection,
analysis, and interpretation of these data, as they relate to our understanding of the
disease process, and the eventual control of exposures that may lead to the induction
of these cancers.

Data on potential chemical exposures involved in the induction of cancer are
available from case reports, reports of the occurrence of clusters of cancers, and
from descriptive and analytic epidemiologic studies, primarily of workers in occupational settings. Reports of clinical cases and clusters of cancers among persons
with a common occupation or exposure generally serve to alert the health community so that epidemiologic research may be pursued. Similarly, cross-sectional
or descriptive epidemiologic studies that have identified patterns of disease distribution over time, in different geographic areas, or related to certain demographic
characteristics, can generate hypotheses about etiologic factors that may be pursued
by analytic studies. The analytic epidemiologic studies used to test causal hypotheses are of two types: case-control studies and cohort studies. The case-control
study is a retrospective case history (100) that compares past exposures of persons
with and without a particular disease. It is most suitable in studies of rare diseases.
The cohort study or prospective, longitudinal, or follow-up study, follows a group
of persons (for example, with the same occupation) forward in time to observe

---

[1]The views expressed are those of the author and do not necessarily represent those of the Occupational Safety and Health Administration.

disease outcome. The advantage of this type of study design is that it permits a direct measure of the incidence or risk of developing a disease in individuals with a specific characteristic or exposure. The advantages and disadvantages of the different epidemiologic study designs in occupational settings have been described in detail by Schottenfeld and Haas (100), by Monson (77), and others. Certain of these will be pointed out in the discussion of individual studies that follows. The data used in this evaluation are largely drawn from occupational epidemiologic studies.

A number of difficulties are associated with a review of the epidemiologic literature concerning chemically induced leukemias and lymphomas. The first concerns the constantly evolving nomenclature and the confusing variety of classification systems being used to describe and define these cancers. Over the years the classifications of the various forms of leukemia or lymphoma have differed widely as new scientific and clinical information on each disease entity has become available and is incorporated. Second, epidemiologists and nosologists have traditionally relied on the International Classification of Diseases (ICD) developed by the World Health Organization (122) to classify disease entities according to a standardized system, thereby making study results comparable. Unfortunately, the ICD cannot keep up with the state of the art for every disease in its system. Third, because cancers are relatively rare events, it is frequently necessary to combine categories in epidemiologic studies in order to have sufficient numbers to permit analysis. Unfortunately, this results in the combining of cancers of many cell types and origins into the so-called lymphohemopoietic system, possibly masking or losing information on differences in etiology. Fourth, diagnosis differs over the years between individuals and between institutions. This may become a significant problem when attempting to follow a cohort of persons employed in a particular industry over a 30-year period. When compiling data on causes of mortality, the assumption must be made that some leukemias will be diagnosed as lymphomas and vice versa and recorded as such on the death certificates.

O'Conor (84) points out that comparisons of tumor incidence in different countries or regions have provided etiologic leads that form the basis for testable hypotheses. However, the validity and utility of these comparisons depend on the accuracy of demographic definitions, reliability of diagnosis, degree of uniformity of nomenclature and classification in data from cancer registries, and vital or other health records. A classification system should have clinical or etiologic relevance. With neoplastic diseases the classification has been based on cellular morphology and histogenesis which relate to prognosis and response to treatment. Classification on an etiologic basis has not been possible. The older systems of classification of lymphoid neoplasms generally included four groups: lymphosarcoma, reticulum cell sarcoma, Hodgkin's disease, and lymphatic leukemia. The eighth revision of the ICD (ICD8) combined lymphosarcoma and reticulum cell sarcoma into one category (ICD8, code 200) leaving Hodgkin's disease (ICD8, code 201) and lymphatic leukemia (ICD8, code 204) to make up the three major categories. O'Conor (84) finds this classification inadequate for clinical or epidemiologic investigations in light of present knowledge of the functional components of the lymphoreticular system. A working classification of non-Hodgkin's lymphoma has been developed for clinical use that can translate to or from existing classifications and that will serve for etiologic studies when ICD-O (121) code numbers have been assigned. It remains to be seen whether this classification will add clarity or further obscure etiologic studies.

Rundles (97) points out that it is important to recognize that most clinical, pathologic, therapeutic, and end-result compilations pertaining to chronic lymphocytic leukemia in the past have included variable numbers of the other related diseases such as lymphosarcoma, T-cell or B-cell leukemias, hairy cell leukemias, and some lymphomas.

Morgan and Banks (81) note that the distinction between lymphoma and lymphoid leukemia is purely distributional, that is, a particular lymphoid neoplasm may manifest both lymphomatous and leukemic features during the course of the disease.

Because certain of the leukemias and lymphomas share diagnostic traits and because of the changes in diagnosis and classification over the years, it is important to examine epidemiologic data from two aspects. The analysis of cancer mortality data using vital records or death certificates should include all related diseases to ensure that diseases of similar etiology that may have been misdiagnosed or misclassified will be included and that useful information will not be lost. However, this may dilute the data too much. Each separate cell type or major disease entity should also be analyzed separately (limited by sample size) to distinguish important differences in target-cell specificity of particular chemical exposures, thus preserving mechanistic information, which varies by disease entity.

In general, the problems of interpretation of data from occupational epidemiologic studies can be included under the following general headings: differences between incidence and mortality rates, ascertainment of disease cases, consistency of diagnosis, ascertainment of exposure (dose and dose rate), misclassification of exposure or diagnosis, identification of population at risk, inclusion of appropriate control or comparison groups, and potential confounding by exposures to other etiologic agents such as radiation and viruses. Many of these problems relate to the design of the study and can be adequately addressed by proper study design. Others often cannot be completely corrected and require use of the best available data. In either case, the better the control of these factors, the firmer the conclusions on etiology that can be derived from these studies.

Incidence and mortality rates for lymphoid and hemopoietic cancers may differ for several reasons. Depending on the case/fatality rate for the particular tumor, mortality data may more or less truly reflect the incidence of the disease in the population. Mortality statistics are usually collected from death certificates filed with centralized authorities. Incidence rates, which count new cases of the disease and not just deaths, are more difficult to estimate and are usually obtained in the United States through population-based disease registries. However, the diagnoses are more likely to be accurate because they are usually based on medical records including pathology reports. Tables 1 and 2 present incidence and mortality rates for lymphoid and hemopoietic cancers for the total U.S. population.

Employment in several occupations has been associated with increases in incidence of or mortality from leukemias or lymphomas in general; persons in these occupations reported to be at increased risk include rubber workers, metal workers, chemical production workers, refinery workers, painters, beauticians, farmers, chemists, and workers in health occupations. Chemical or chemical mixture exposures reported to be associated with increases in incidence of or mortality from leukemias or lymphomas include exposures through occupation or medical treatment to benzene, styrene, 1,3-butadiene, ethylene oxide, vinyl chloride, polychlorinated biphenyls, pesticides, toluene, paint, nitrites, chemotherapeutic agents, antibiotics, anti-inflammatory drugs, and lithium. The data vary in the quality of information provided about etiology of these cancers. The major studies or groups of studies are considered here under each disease entity.

LEUKEMIA

The term leukemia applies to "a diverse group of malignancies that share in common merely the fact that all arise from cell systems that circulate in peripheral blood and that arise in large part from bone marrow" (47). The epidemiology of leukemia has been reviewed by Alderson (11), Heath (47), and others (13,65). Chemical etiologies for leukemia, with the exception of benzene, are not, in general, well documented in the epidemiologic literature. Several reasons for this may be

TABLE 1. Annual age-adjusted incidence rates per 100,000 persons in the United States for 1969–1971 by race[a]

	Incidence per 100,000	
Cancer site	White	Black
All sites	297.7	318.8
Total chronic leukemia:	5.4	4.9
Chronic lymphocytic	3.0	2.5
Chronic granulocytic	2.0	1.7
Lymphosarcoma and reticulum cell sarcoma	4.9	3.3
Total acute leukemia:	4.5	3.1
Acute lymphocytic	1.2	0.7
Acute granulocytic	2.4	1.7
Monocytic	0.4	0.2
Multiple myeloma	3.3	7.2
Hodgkin's disease	3.4	2.1
Other forms of lymphoma	1.8	1.4

[a]Incidence rates adjusted to 1970 standard population of the United States.
Source: Cutler and Young (26).

TABLE 2. *Average annual age-adjusted mortality rates per 100,000 persons in the United States, 1960–1969 and 1970–1979 by race and gender[a]*

| Cancer site (ICD 9th revision) | White | | | | Nonwhite | | | |
| | Male | | Female | | Male | | Female | |
	60–69	70–79	60–69	70–79	60–69	70–79	60–69	70–79
All cancers	190.0	204.1	132.4	131.7	209.5	231.6	142.3	133.1
Lymphosarcoma and reticulum cell sarcoma, including other lymphoma (200,202, 159.1,202.0,202.1, 202.8,202.9)	5.6	6.0	3.7	4.1	3.8	3.8	2.1	2.2
Hodgkin's disease (201)	2.3	1.6	1.4	1.0	1.7	1.1	0.8	0.5
Multiple myeloma (203 except 203.1)	2.1	2.7	1.5	1.8	3.4	4.6	2.2	3.1
Leukemias (204–208,202.4,203.1)	9.5	9.1	5.9	5.4	6.3	6.4	4.1	4.0

[a]Total U.S. age-specific population for 1970 used as the standard.
Source: Riggan et al. (93).

suggested: (a) incidence and mortality statistics are generally listed by major cell types that are most frequently occurring; (b) some of these cell types may be grouped because of small numbers of cases; (c) mortality statistics rely on proper listing on death certificates; (d) differential diagnosis may be difficult or incorrect (misclassification); (e) mortality statistics derived from death certificates provide little or no information on occupation or exposure.

Increased risk of leukemia has been associated with various occupations, including painting in the construction industry, rubber product manufacture, shoe manufacture, rotogravure printing, farming, medical product manufacture, and others. A number of chemical exposures might have been important in the etiology of these cancers, but benzene occurs with the greatest frequency in a number of these occupations, as can be seen in Table 3. Chemical or biologic agents suspected of involvement in the etiology of leukemias have also included ethylene oxide (48,49), solvents (24), antineoplastic agents and other drugs (2), and infectious organisms (99). The association between exposure to ionizing radiation and leukemia is well established (25,47,65).

The epidemiologic evidence to support the causal association between benzene exposure and myelogenous leukemia is extensive and is further supported by numerous case reports describing leukemia in workers exposed to benzene. Moreover, benzene exposure, alone or combined with other chemicals, has been associated with monocytic leukemia, acute and chronic lymphatic leukemia, multiple myeloma, and various forms of lymphoma.

Aksoy and co-workers in Turkey (4–9) and Vigliani and co-workers in Italy (116–118) have reported a series of cases of myelogenous, monocytic, erythroblastic, and lymphocytic leukemia, aplastic anemia, pancytopenia, lymphoma, Hodg-

TABLE 3. Studies indicating increased risk of lymphohemopoietic cancers in occupations with potential benzene exposure

Occupation	Cancer site(s) reported	Type of study	Reference
"Benzene risk" occupations	Acute myeloblastic leukemia	Case control	(103)
Occupations using benzene or coal tar fractions	Reticulum cell sarcoma; lymphosarcoma; Hodgkin's disease	Case control	(115)
Chemical manufacturing	Myelogenous leukemia	Historical prospective cohort mortality	(90)
	Leukemia; multiple myeloma	Historical prospective cohort mortality	(28)
	Leukemia; acute myelogenous leukemia	Historical prospective cohort mortality	(Shell, unpubl.)
	Chronic myeloid leukemia; chronic lymphatic leukemia; acute lymphatic leukemia; unspecified lymphatic leukemia; acute unspecified leukemia; multiple myeloma; reticulum cell sarcoma; Hodgkin's disease; lymphosarcoma; other lymphoid tissue neoplasms	Historical prospective cohort mortality	(Wong, unpubl.)
Chemical handling	Hodgkin's disease	Case control	(88)
Chemists	Lymphohemopoietic neoplasms; lymphoma; leukemia	Proportional mortality	(63,102)
	Lymphoma, leukemia; Hodgkin's disease; lymphosarcoma; acute myelogenous leukemia; chronic myelogenous leukemia; reticulum cell sarcoma	Historical prospective cohort mortality	(85–87)

Pathologists	Lymphohemopoietic neoplasms other than Hodgkin's or leukemia	Historical prospective cohort mortality	(45)
Petroleum industry: Refinery workers	Lymphocytic leukemia	Prospective cohort morbidity & mortality	(101)
Petrochemical workers	Multiple myeloma	Prospective cohort morbidity & mortality	(101)
Petroleum products with exposure to motor fuel	Acute nonlymphocytic leukemia	Case control	(19)
Refinery work	Leukemia; multiple myeloma; Hodgkin's disease; non-Hodgkin's lymphoma	Proportional mortality	(107,109)
	Leukemia	Case control	(98)
	Leukemia; Hodgkin's disease; lymphopoietic cancers	Historical prospective cohort mortality	(120)
Rubber hydrochloride manufacture	Myelogenous or monocytic leukemia	Historical prospective cohort mortality	(52,94)
Rubber industry	Leukemia; chronic lymphatic leukemia; lymphocytic leukemia; myelogenous leukemia; lymphosarcoma; lymphoma	Proportional mortality, historical prospective cohort mortality, and case control	(12,24,29,69, 70–72,78,79, 112)
Shoe manufacturing	Myelogenous, monocytic, erythroblastic and lymphocytic leukemia; non-Hodgkin's lymphoma; Hodgkin's disease; multiple myeloma	Case series	(4–9)
Shoe manufacturing; rotogravure industry	Leukemia	Case series	(116–118)
With exposure to organic solvents, chlorophenols, phenoxy acids	Lymphoma; Hodgkin's disease	Case control	(44)

kin's disease, and multiple myeloma among workers occupationally exposed to benzene in shoe manufacturing, rotogravure printing, and other industries.

Because of the need to follow these case reports with a comprehensive epidemiologic investigation, the National Institute for Occupational Safety and Health (NIOSH) initiated a study of a cohort of workers exposed to benzene in the manufacture of rubber hydrochloride. An unusual pattern of mortality found during the course of the study stimulated the authors to report the results of the cohort mortality study with 75% completion of vital status follow-up (52). Among 748 white male employees exposed to benzene between 1940 and 1949 and followed through 1975, there were 7 deaths from myelogenous or monocytic leukemia compared with an expected number of 1.38 leukemia deaths for U.S. white males of similar age and during a similar calendar period. The standardized mortality ratio (SMR) (SMR = observed/expected × 100) was 506, and excess mortality due to these leukemias was significant ($p < 0.002$). Monitoring data and industrial hygiene assessments led to the conclusion that the working environment of this cohort was not contaminated with other materials known to induce blood dyscrasias.

Rinsky et al. (94) completed the follow-up of this group of employees. They found 7 cases of leukemia compared with 1.25 expected, resulting in an SMR of 560. Because 58% of the cohort members had been employed for less than 1 year, the data were analyzed by length of employment. Five of the leukemia deaths occurred in workers employed 5 or more years, compared with 0.23 expected (SMR = 2,100). Five additional cases of leukemia, 4 of them myelogenous, were reported among workers in these rubber hydrochloride manufacturing facilities. However, these 5 could not be included in the statistical analysis for this study because they did not fit the strict cohort definition. Rinsky et al. (94) described in detail the historical and industrial hygiene data on benzene exposure levels at these two plants from all available sources. They concluded on the basis of the data that exposure to benzene was generally within the recommended occupational exposure limits at the time of exposure.

The NIOSH study has been discussed repeatedly, with particular attention to the estimation of past benzene exposure levels associated with the induction of leukemia in those workers (53–55,106). This has resulted in a thorough reexamination of the data on which the authors based their conclusions. Infante and co-workers (55) recently responded to further questions relating to estimated exposure levels used for a leukemia-risk assessment. They concluded,

> We believe that the actual exposure levels to individual workers comprising the NIOSH study will never be known precisely. However, much effort has been made to characterize their exposure, resulting in reasonable estimates that are better in quality and in detail than for most historical prospective occupational mortality studies.

The estimation of past exposure levels to carcinogens and other toxic materials in the occupational setting continues to spark controversy for scientific, economic, and political reasons. In establishing cause and effect relationships in the ideal situation, one has available precise measurements of the concentrations of a variety of chemicals in a variety of occupational situations. When studying chronic diseases, such as cancer, in which there is a relatively long period of time between the initial exposure and recognition of disease, it would be optimal if those precise measurements were available for situations spanning 30 or 40 years into the past. However, it is unlikely that such detailed information will be available, and in the case of the NIOSH study, such detailed exposure data are not available. It is then necessary to make reasonable assumptions using all available information, including results of exposure measurements, descriptions of analytic methods utilized in the past, historical data on processes, work practices, etc. The NIOSH investigators made a reconstruction of exposures based on fairly extensive exposure data at one facility (more than 100 measurements), some exposure data at the other facility, and contemporaneous reports indicating that respirators generally were worn when exposures were over the recommended limit.

Ott et al. (90) conducted a historical prospective mortality study of 594 white males occupationally exposed to benzene who had been employed in a chemical manufacturing facility at any time between 1940 and 1970. Three cases of myelogenous leukemia were observed, whereas 0.8 were expected based on incidence data from the Third National Cancer Survey. The excess was statistically significant. Also, 1 death from aplastic anemia and 1 death from pernicious anemia were observed in this cohort.

Decoufle et al. (28) reported on a historical prospective cohort mortality study of 259 male employees who were employed from January 1, 1947, through December 31, 1960, at a chemical plant where benzene had been used in large quantities. By December 31, 1977, 4 deaths from lymphoreticular cancers had occurred when 1.1 would have been expected, based on the national rate. This resulted in a relative risk (RR) of 3.7. Three of the deaths were due to leukemia as compared to 0.4 expected, resulting in a relative risk of 6.8. One of the persons who died from leukemia had begun treatment for multiple myeloma 2 years prior to his development of leukemia. The authors noted that the 2-year latency period from initiation of chemotherapy to development of leukemia in this case was typical of that seen in other instances of therapy-induced leukemia in myeloma patients. The expected number of deaths from multiple myeloma was estimated by the first author to be 0.23 (27). The 2 cases of multiple myeloma observed in the study plus previous reports of multiple myeloma associated with benzene exposure suggested to the authors an etiologic role for benzene in the pathologies of tumors of B-cell lineage (multiple myeloma and chronic lymphatic leukemia). The authors did not present any information on benzene exposure levels for these chemical workers.

Several epidemiologic studies of refinery workers have reported excesses of deaths due to lymphoid and hemopoietic cancers. Thomas et al. (107) examined the cause-specific mortality experience of 3,105 members of the Oil, Chemical and Atomic Workers International Union (OCAW). Deaths among active union members in Texas between 1947 and 1977 were identified through membership records, and their death certificates were obtained. Among other cancer excesses reported by these authors, increased relative frequencies of leukemia (ICD 8th

Revision 204-207) and multiple myeloma (ICD8, 203) were observed among white male refinery and petrochemical plant workers who had been union members for 10 or more years. The authors noted that the observation of increasing cancer risks with longer union membership strengthens the possibility of an association with occupational factors such as benzene and other petrochemicals.

Because increased frequencies of cancer deaths were found for union members who had been employed at these three refineries, and because the original data were limited to active union members, Thomas et al. (109) added deaths among retired union members to assemble a more complete data set and focused their study on the cause-specific mortality for 2,509 active and retired members of the OCAW. Combining data for the three refineries, deaths due to hemopoietic and lymphoid cancers [proportionate mortality ratio (PMR) = 161], leukemia (PMR = 183), multiple myeloma (PMR = 196), Hodgkin's disease (PMR = 134), and non-Hodgkin's lymphoma (PMR = 132) were elevated, with significant excesses of leukemia, multiple myeloma, and Hodgkin's disease among retired workers. Deaths from cancer of the brain, prostate, stomach, pancreas, and skin were also significantly elevated.

Following the previous cohort mortality studies, Thomas et al. (108) conducted a case-control study that examined work histories for evidence of any unusual distributions by work category to evaluate the increased risk of mortality from brain tumors, stomach cancer, leukemia, and other cancers found in the proportionate mortality analysis among OCAW members who had been employed at these three Texas oil refineries. Work histories were obtained from company personnel records and summarized by classifying job titles and departments into work categories. A worker was exposed to a work category if he had worked at least 1 day in that category 15 or more years prior to his death. Controls were selected from active and retired union members who had worked at the same refinery, were of the same race and sex, and had died of causes other than those being investigated. Cases and controls were matched on age at death, date of death, and date of first membership in the union. Additional cases identified subsequent to the proportionate mortality study and added to the data from that study included 1 brain tumor, 4 stomach cancers, and 4 leukemia cases. One leukemia case was eliminated because the wrong death certificate was obtained, and work histories were not located for 2 leukemia cases, leaving 34 leukemia cases in the analysis. Controls used for brain tumor, stomach cancer, and leukemia comparisons were pooled, and their work histories were used to estimate usual employment patterns within refinery work categories. These "usual" patterns were compared with work histories of the 9 cases of multiple myeloma, 9 cases of Hodgkin's disease, and 23 cases of non-Hodgkin's lymphoma identified in the previous PMR study.

Maximum likelihood estimates of the relative risk (odds ratio) for leukemia and other cancers for each work category were calculated. Odds ratios for leukemia were elevated only among persons exposed to two categories: treating and boilermaking. For these two categories the risk of leukemia increased with increasing duration of employment. In the comparisons with pooled controls, no unusual distributions with work category were noted for the cases of multiple myeloma, Hodgkin's disease, or non-Hodgkin's lymphoma. These investigators noted that their work categories may not be true indicators of exposure because there was potential for contact with many substances within a category and workers may have had contact with the same substance in more than one category. Because of job mobility, many workers were classified as exposed in several work categories. However, there was very little overlap of exposure to treating and boilermaking categories among leukemia cases and controls. The number of cases of each cancer type was small; consequently, the ability to detect excess risk was low unless the actual risk was very high. All of the comparisons were made between persons who had worked at refineries so that general occupational exposures may have caused them to be indistinguishable. During treating, petroleum products are refined and combined with additives. Benzene exposure is, however, not category specific; perhaps this accounts for the lack of a strong association for leukemia with any specific job category. As indicated previously, because they examined risks for a number of cancers, exposure was defined as at least 1 day of work in a category at least 15 years prior to death. At first glance one might worry that this would exclude exposures that were important in the development of cancers with a shorter latency period, such as leukemia. The authors stated, however, that changing the definition of exposure "by eliminating the latency period did not alter the results."

In a preliminary report of a prospective study of the morbidity and mortality of petroleum industry employees in the United States, Schottenfeld et al. (101) observed statistically significant increases in the incidence of acute and chronic lymphocytic leukemias among refinery workers and of multiple myeloma among petrochemical workers. Expected values were derived from U.S. age-specific cancer incidence rates from the Surveillance, Epidemiology, and End Results (SEER) program of the National Cancer Institute for 1977. Seven cases of acute and chronic lymphocytic leukemias were observed among refinery workers compared with 2.6 expected for a standardized incidence ratio (SIR) of 274. Nonlymphocytic leukemias were increased in petrochemical and refinery workers (SIR = 113), but not significantly. Multiple myeloma was elevated significantly among the petrochemical workers (SIR = 552). The authors stated that these results should be viewed as preliminary because the period of observation was quite short, the number of older workers included in the analysis was limited, and the degree of underreporting of mortality was unknown. In view of the comments by Blattner (17), regarding the increasing frequency of multiple myeloma with age, one would expect that the SIR would be likely to increase as follow-up of these workers continues.

Rushton and Alderson (98) reported the results of a case-control study of leukemia deaths among men employed at eight oil refineries in the United Kingdom. Two sets of controls were selected from the total refinery population: one was matched with cases by refinery and year of birth, the other matched by refinery, year of birth, and length of service. Job histories obtained from refinery personnel records were used to categorize each person's benzene exposure as low, medium, or high, and the potential benzene exposure of cases was compared with that of controls. Although no overall excess of deaths from leukemia was found when compared with expected numbers based on national rates, the risk of leukemia for men with medium or high exposure was significantly greater ($p = 0.05$) than the risk for men with low benzene exposure.

Tsai et al. (111) found no statistically significant increases in mortality from lymphoid and hemopoietic cancers among Texas refinery workers. No deaths from leukemia or lymphohemopoietic cancers were observed among 34 deceased employees identified as having worked in benzene areas at any time between September 1952 and January 1978.

Wen et al. (120) studied male hourly and salaried workers employed for any length of time at a refinery in Port Arthur, Texas, between January 1937 and January 1978. Although these authors found no statistically significant increases in mortality (except for bone cancer) among these workers compared with the general U.S. population, nonsignificant increases in SMRs were observed for Hodgkin's disease, leukemia, cancer of other lymphatic tissue (ICDA8, 208), kidney, and skin cancers. Furthermore, nonsignificant excesses were noted in deaths due to leukemia among white hourly workers, Hodgkin's disease and cancer of other lymphatic tissue among nonwhite hourly workers, and lymphopoietic cancers among salaried workers.

The study by Wen et al. has been criticized by other investigators (51,62,82) because the cohort was made up of all Gulf employees and thus included many unexposed persons in the population at risk, including clerical and managerial employees. Because Wen et al. did not identify the population at risk of exposure to the refinery process, the SMRs might have been diluted, resulting in the non-statistically significant excesses in deaths for lymphoid and hemopoietic or other cancers. Moreover, because 9% to 10% (338 deaths) of the cohort was lost to follow-up, with more complete follow-up the SMRs might increase. Those lost to follow-up may have included terminated employees with possibly shorter durations of exposure.

In 1983 the Shell Oil Company (*unpublished report*, OSHA Docket #H-059, Exhibit #142-13A) reported results of a mortality study among active employees and retirees from two manufacturing locations. Deaths occurred between January 1, 1973, and December 31, 1982. At one facility, a significant excess of deaths due to leukemia was observed (14 observed; 6.4 expected), resulting in a SMR of 219 for all leukemias. Eight deaths were observed from acute myelogenous leukemia (AML) whereas 2.0 were expected, resulting in a SMR of 400. At the second facility, 6 deaths from all forms of leukemia were noted among refinery workers as compared with 2.6 expected (SMR = 230). Three acute myelogenous leukemia deaths were observed versus approximately 0.8 expected (SMR = 375). These results were of borderline statistical significance. The study of mortality at both of these facilities examined causes of death for "active" employees and retirees and excluded "terminees" who were not followed after termination of employment at Shell. Thus, the actual number of cases of leukemia related to exposure in this occupational setting may have been greater.

A historical prospective mortality study was conducted by Wong et al. (1983; *unpublished report*, OSHA Docket #H-059, Exhibit #151A) for the Chemical Manufacturers Association (CMA). The mortality experience of 4,602 male chemical workers from seven plants who were occupationally exposed to benzene for at least 6 months between 1946 and 1975 was compared with that of 3,074 chemical workers from the same or similar plants who had no known occupational exposure to benzene. Vital status was followed through December 31, 1977. Of the 7,676 men in the total cohort, 6,463 (84.2%) were found to be alive, 1,036 (13.5%) were deceased, and 177 (2.3%) were of unknown vital status. Death certificates were obtained for 1,013 (97.8%) of the deceased employees. Those lost to follow-up were included in the analysis only until the last date of contact, and their mortality experience was assumed to be similar to the rest of the cohort.

Exposure to benzene was divided into continuous (with some intermittent) exposure (3,536 men) and intermittent or casual exposure (1,066 men). Each job was divided into 34 uniform tasks and the amount of time spent at each task was determined. Benzene exposure for each task was estimated, based on available industrial hygiene measurements and historical data. These were summed for each job.

The SMR was used to compare cause-specific mortality for both those exposed and unexposed to benzene with the general U.S. population. Expected values were based on U.S. national age-cause-race-specific mortality rates for 5-year time periods from 1946 to 1977. For some site-specific cancers that appeared to be in excess among the benzene-exposed cohort, further analyses were conducted contrasting observed deaths in the exposed group with observed deaths among workers at the same plants who were not exposed to benzene.

Age- and race-adjusted Mantel-Haenszel chi-squares and relative risks for all lymphoid and hemopoietic cancers combined indicated a significantly increased risk for benzene-exposed (continuous and intermittent) white males ($RR = 4.66$, $p = 0.03$) when compared with the nonexposed workers. This excess was primarily due to 7 leukemia deaths observed in the exposed group, whereas none were observed in the nonexposed group. When only continuously benzene-exposed workers were compared with the nonexposed group, the excess of lymphohemopoietic cancer was significant for white males and all males, respectively ($RR = 5.3$, $p = 0.02$; $RR = 3.2$, $p = 0.04$). None of the 7 leukemia deaths were of the acute myelogenous cell type. Two were chronic myeloid leukemia, 2 were chronic lymphatic leukemia, and 1 each was from unspecified lymphatic leukemia, acute lymphatic leukemia, and acute other unspecified leukemia. The remaining lymphoid and hemopoietic cancer deaths in benzene-exposed workers were due to: multiple myeloma, 3; reticulum cell sarcoma, 3; Hodgkin's disease, 2; lymphosarcoma, 1; and other lymphoid tissue neoplasms, 3.

Of the 3 deaths from multiple myeloma observed among the benzene-exposed workers, 2 were identified among the intermittent exposure group as compared with 0.56 expected ($RR = 3.8$) based on U.S. rates. Because deaths from multiple myeloma were not observed among the nonbenzene-exposed workers, an expected value based on the latter group would not have been appropriate.

When the data were analyzed by cumulative exposure, statistically significant dose-response relationships were detected for leukemia as well as for the broader category of all lymphopoietic cancer. For those with less than 180 ppm-months of exposure, a twofold increased risk of all lymphohematopoietic cancers was observed, whereas for those with more than 720 ppm-months of benzene exposure, a fourfold relative risk of all lymphoid and hemopoietic cancers combined was observed when compared with the mortality experience of nonbenzene-exposed employees. The Mantel-Haenszel chi-square was significant for an upward trend analysis for all lymphoid and hemopoietic cancers (ICD8, 200-209) ($p = 0.02$) and for leukemia (ICD8, 204-207) ($p = 0.01$) and of borderline significance ($p = 0.057$) for non-Hodgkin's lymphopoietic cancer (ICD8, 200, 202-207). As a result of these analyses, Wong et al. concluded that there was a significant association between occupational exposure to benzene and leukemia, all lymphopoietic cancers, as well as non-Hodgkin's lymphoma.

Thorpe (110) reviewed data for 38,000 petroleum-refining and petrochemical workers in eight European countries. He reported no excess of deaths due to leukemia. IARC reviewed his study and stated "the study suffers from problems of ascertainment, specificity and validity of diagnosis and the 'healthy worker effect' in the calculation of SMRs" (57). More detailed discussions of the limitations of the methodology used by Thorpe have been published (20,57,54).

A number of studies have noted excesses of mortality from chronic lymphatic leukemia, myelogenous leukemia, and lymphosarcoma among persons exposed to benzene and benzene-containing solvents while employed in the rubber industry (12,29,72,79,112).

In a study involving 784 persons who were employed in a rubber plant in Finland for at least 3 months between 1953 and 1976 and followed from January 1, 1953, to December 21, 1976, Kilpikari (60,61) reported no significant excess cancer risk. However, the number of workers studied was quite small, the follow-up period was short, and the deaths were few, resulting in little statistical power to detect an increase in risk, if one were present.

The International Agency for Research on Cancer (IARC) has reviewed many of the epidemiologic studies relating occupational exposures in the rubber industry to increased risk of cancer (56). In follow-up studies of rubber workers in the United States and in one study in the United Kingdom, excess mortality from lymphoid and hemopoietic cancers has been reported. In the United States three major populations of rubber workers have been studied. In one of these, the excess of leukemia was highest in workers in compounding and mixing jobs, tire inspection, and in synthetic rubber manufacture (70). The leukemia excess in synthetic workers was due to lymphatic leukemia. In another U.S. group, an excess of leukemia was highest among workers in calendaring, tire building, and tire-curing operations (78). Excesses of lymphomas were also found among U.S. rubber workers. A case-control study of lymphatic and hematopoietic cancers in the population of rubber workers from seven U.S. plants showed an increased risk of lymphatic leukemia (RR = 3.3) for workers in jobs with exposure to solvents (72).

The IARC workgroup (56) suggested that the excess of malignancies of the lymphoid and hemopoietic systems among U.S. rubber workers may have resulted from exposure to benzene that was used in the past as a solvent and may be a contaminant of organic solvents used at present. Furthermore, many materials that are present in the work atmospheres in the rubber industry, in addition to benzene, have been found to be mutagenic or carcinogenic in experimental systems. The combination of chemical exposures in the rubber industry increases the likelihood of effects of interaction between these agents and between these agents and non-occupational factors. On the basis of the quality of the epidemiologic studies reviewed and the strength and consistency of the reported cancer associations within the rubber industry, the IARC reviewers found that there was sufficient evidence to support a causal association between excess leukemias and occupational exposures, presumably to solvents, in the rubber industry. The data on lymphoma indicated an excess occurrence in rubber workers but were not adequate to support a causal association with occupational exposures.

Because of the associations between leukemia and solvent exposure found in earlier studies, Checkoway et al. (24) conducted a case-control study of lymphocytic leukemia. They found that exposure in the rubber industry to a number of solvents, including carbon tetrachloride, carbon disulfide, and benzene, was associated with increased risk of this cancer.

MULTIPLE MYELOMA

Multiple myeloma is a malignancy of plasma cells usually arising in the bone marrow. Multiple myeloma is relatively easy to diagnose, but it was classified as a bone tumor until 1949 when the ICD included it in the lymphoid and hemopoietic neoplasms. The epidemiology of multiple myeloma has been reviewed by Agu et al. (3), Blattner (17), and Blattner et al. (18). Agu et al. (3) examined age- and race-adjusted mortality rates for multiple myeloma in 31 Texas state economic areas (TSEA) for which demographic and occupational information was available. A significant ($p < 0.05$) positive association was found, with percentage of the population in each TSEA employed in beauty shops, carpentry, and agricultural industries. Blattner et al. (18) combined mortality rates for groups of U.S. counties in state economic areas (SEA). For the years 1950 to 1975, multiple myeloma mortality rates were elevated for white males in SEAs with high petroleum and paper production and furniture manufacturing.

Guidotti et al. (40) analyzed data from a population-based cancer registry for Los Angeles County by occupation and industry. An excess in the number of cases of multiple myeloma was reported for females in the occupation "cosmetologists, hairdressers, and manicurists."

These analyses of incidence or mortality data are useful in the development of etiologic hypotheses using information available from vital statistics compilations and cancer registries. They can provide important clues to etiology through descriptions of the distribution of disease in a population and the delineation of differential disease rates among segments of the population according to demographic, geographic, or other characteristics including occupation. However, the precision of these types of studies is low and they must be followed up with analytic studies of cohorts of persons in an occupation that include examinations of potential etiologic agents that are present in that particular occupational setting. An evaluation of information on cancer induction from experimental studies in other species and from epidemiologic studies in other industries with similar chemical exposures or in the same industry with different chemical exposures can add valuable clues to the study of causality.

For example, Guidotti et al. (40) found no cases of multiple myeloma among barbers in their data base, although the number of cancer cases was small and suggested that chemical exposures to barbers may be different than those of cosmetologists. They compared their results with those of another investigator who reported excesses of multiple myeloma among cosmetologists and barbers using a similar ecologic study design (74) and with those of an investigator who found no excess risk of cancer of any site among male British hairdressers and barbers (10). They then reviewed the possible chemical exposures for cosmetologists, hairdressers, and manicurists, for example, in dyes, shampoos, conditioners, permanent wave solutions, etc., listed those with known mutagenic or carcinogenic potential, and pointed to the need for further study of specific chemical exposures.

Blattner (17) concluded that numerous clinical and epidemiologic reports suggest that occupational exposures may induce myeloma, but he found these observations to be preliminary. The exposure or occupational risk factors for multiple myeloma he found in a survey of the literature included radiation; farming; heavy metals (lead, arsenic, copper); asbestos; petrochemicals, refining, plastics, and/or rubber industries; furniture and wood-related industries; leather workers; food handlers, processors, kitchen workers; and a number of miscellaneous occupational groups. He found it difficult to isolate particular chemical risk factors for multiple myeloma among these occupations. He suggested that investigators who do not follow workers through life are likely to miss myeloma because of its increasing association with age and of the fact that it is a rare neoplasm. He concluded that further studies are needed to evaluate leads to environmental exposures and immunogenetic factors, stating that some agents may act through antigenic stimulation or suppression of immunoregulatory function. Furthermore, any clarification of the causes and mechanisms of multiple myeloma will require an integration of epidemiologic studies of high-risk populations and basic research into the normal process of B-cell ontogeny and the factors regulating this process.

NON-HODGKIN'S LYMPHOMA

Greene (35) and Mack and Preston-Martin (65) reviewed the epidemiology of non-Hodgkin's lymphoma (NHL). This category is reserved for all lymphomas remaining after Hodgkin's disease; plasma cell neoplasms and Burkitt's lymphoma have been excluded. It therefore represents an extremely heterogeneous group of lymphoreticular neoplasms. Greene (35) notes the difficulty of evaluating occupational factors involved in NHL when, for most studies, NHL is combined with other lymphoid and hemopoietic neoplasms. He reviewed six surveys of occupation and cancer and found excesses of lymphoma reported among sales and clerical personnel, postal workers, insurance and real estate brokers, engineers, electrical workers, mechanics, machinists, primary metal workers, and farmers. He noted that some of these occupational groups may reflect socioeconomic or environmental factors or chemical/physical exposures at the workplace. For example, the association of NHL with some electrical occupations may be related to exposure to high-current flow electrical fields. Reports for some occupational groups have been inconsistent, particularly those for anesthesiologists and vinyl chloride workers. Chemists show an excess of lymphoma but the specific exposures involved have not been identified. Similarly, rubber workers in tire-building processes show excesses of NHL. Workers in petroleum refining, processing arsenic-containing ore, and exposed to herbicides also show excesses of NHL. Greene finds these to be preliminary indications that occupational chemical exposures may induce NHL.

Vianna and Polan (115) observed a significant excess of deaths due to lymphoma (reticulum cell sarcoma, lymphosarcoma, and Hodgkin's disease) in men employed in occupations where benzene and/or coal tar fractions that may contain benzene were used. All deaths reported to the New York State Department of Health Office of Vital Records, between 1950 and 1969, among men at least 20 years of age who were employed in 14 occupations where benzene exposure might have occurred were tabulated. Crude death rates were calculated using 1960 census data for the benzene-exposed group and compared with rates for residents of New York State, yielding relative risks of 1.6 for reticulum cell sarcoma, 2.1 for lymphosarcoma, and 1.6 for Hodgkin's disease (HD). Age-adjusted rates were calculated for 7 of the 14 exposed occupations. It was not stated which of the 14 were included in this analysis. However, the relative risk for each of the lymphomas was the same or greater than in the crude analysis and the increase in risk was among exposed persons 45 years or older. Enterline (31) criticized this study for the following reasons: Death rates calculated by Vianna and Polan (115) used occupational data from the U.S. census (current or last occupation) and from death certificates (usual occupation). For retired persons, mortality data are not usually reported by occupation. The excess death rates reported are for occupations that Enterline felt were more likely to be usual than current or last, thus possibly inflating the exposed group's death rates. He suggested that Vianna and Polan use PMRs because they are based only on occupation as defined on death certificates to see if the excess mortality from lymphomas disappears.

Smith and Lickiss (103) had reservations about the methods used by Vianna and Polan (115) but attempted to confirm their findings using data on all new cases of NHL (n = 192) and HD (n = 71), diagnosed between 1972 and 1979 in Tasmania. They found no association of NHL and HD with a history of benzene-related occupations (same as those defined by Vianna and Polan) using the Tasmanian State population as control. They repeated the analysis, examining occupational histories of men with acute myeloblastic leukemia, and found a significantly increased risk among men in occupations with potential benzene exposures.

Harrington and Shannon (45) observed excess deaths from lymphoid and hemopoietic neoplasms other than HD or leukemia among English male pathologists (8 observed versus 3.3 expected, $p < 0.01$). Membership lists of professional organizations were used to establish the populations studied. Death records of deceased pathologists who had been on membership lists between 1955 and 1973 and medical laboratory technicians who had been members between August 1963 and December 31, 1973, were obtained. All of the death certificates of the technicians and 97% of those of the pathologists were obtained to ascertain cause of death. The SMRs were calculated by comparison with mortality figures for all medical practitioners and all laboratory technicians from the British registrar general. The authors stated that the excess of lymphomas in this group of pathologists, presumably, could not be explained by factors other than occupation.

To evaluate the cancer experience of chemists, Li et al. (63) examined the mortality experience of 3,637 members of the American Chemical Society who died between 1948 and 1967. Male chemists who died between the ages of 20 and 64 had a significantly higher proportion of deaths due to cancer than did professional men ($p < 0.001$). Among chemists there were 94 deaths due to lymphoid and hemopoietic cancers (ICD7, 200-205) compared with 59 expected ($p < 0.001$) based on age-adjusted relative frequencies of causes of death among 9,957 U.S. professional men who died between ages 20 and 64 in 1950. There were 61 deaths due to malignant lymphoma (ICD7, 200-203,205) compared with 34 expected ($p < 0.001$). There were 33 deaths due to leukemia (ICD7, 204) compared with 25 expected, but this excess was not statistically significant. The lymphoma deaths showed no preponderance of a particular cell type. Among male chemists over age 64 there were 250 cancer deaths compared with 218 expected based on the age-adjusted relative frequency of specific causes of death among all U.S. white males over age 64 in 1959. In this group, there were 33 lymphoid and hemopoietic cancer deaths compared with 17 expected ($p < 0.001$), 17 deaths from malignant lymphomas compared with 8 expected ($p < 0.01$), and 16 deaths from leukemia compared with 9 expected ($p < 0.05$).

The study group was made up of 4,644 American Chemical Society (ACS) members whose deaths were reported to the Society by relatives, colleagues, or employers and whose obituary notices were published in *Chemical and Engineering News* between April 1948 and July 1967. Death certificates were obtained from state health departments for 3,637 (78%) of these ACS members. This method was used to identify persons whose education qualified them for membership in a professional organization of chemists to avoid discrepancies in reporting of occupation on death certificates and census questionnaires. Unfortunately, this method would be likely to introduce bias resulting from self-selection for membership and for the reporting of deaths to the Society. For 71% of the decedents the occupation was listed on the death certificate as chemist, teacher, engineer, or scientist; 29% were usually administrators or managers in the chemical industry. Membership in the ACS was based on possession of a college degree in chemistry or a closely related field. The authors pointed out several biases that might have influenced the results. Nevertheless, in view of the observation of increased frequency of certain cancers in both younger and older age groups, they concluded that the study suggests that occupational exposure may increase the risk of lymphoma and pancreatic cancer among chemists. They were not able to identify particular factors in a chemist's occupation other than exposure to chemicals that have been implicated as carcinogens.

Searle et al. (102) reported preliminary results of a retrospective study of the mortality of British chemists. Death certificates were obtained to ascertain causes of death for 1,332 members of the Royal Institute of Chemistry who died between 1965 and 1975. The proportion of deaths from neoplasms was higher than expected in persons who were aged 36 to 50 years. Among chemists deaths due to lymphoma were also reported to be elevated compared with expected. Further details of the study design were not given in the report.

Olin (87) reported results of a mortality study of 530 men who were graduated from the School of Chemical Engineering at the Royal Institute of Technology, Stockholm, Sweden, between 1930 and 1950. Average age at graduation was 24.6 years. The vital status of 517 persons at the end of 1974 was traced. For the remaining 13 (2.5%) no information was available. Of 517 chemistry graduates, 58 had died compared with 67 expected based on Swedish general mortality rates. Death certificates for the 58 deceased chemists indicated that 22 deaths were attributed to malignant neoplasms compared with 13 expected. Six deaths were due to malignant lymphomas or leukemias (ICD8, 200-207), whereas only 1.7 deaths due to these diseases would have been expected. Three of these deaths were due to HD (ICD8, 201). A senior chemistry professor, who taught at the school since the mid-1930s, divided the group of chemistry graduates into those persons who had done any sort of laboratory work after graduation and those who had not. Individuals who had done laboratory work numbered 408; those who had not numbered 109. The two groups were similar in age-distribution and general death rates, but 21 of the 22 cancer deaths had occurred among the laboratory group ($p<0.002$). Out of 9 chemists who had died from leukemia/lymphoma or neoplasms of the urinary organs, 8 were classified as organic chemists.

Olin (85) followed a similar group of chemistry graduates from the Chalmers Institute of Technology, Gothenburg, Sweden. They also were graduated between 1930 and 1950 and were followed until the end of 1974. The groups were combined, giving a total cohort of 857 chemistry graduates from the two schools of whom 93 had died. The significant increases in deaths from all cancers, leukemias, lymphomas, and urogenital tumors, compared with expected rates from the general Swedish population, that were found in the first study persisted. Leukemias and lymphomas accounted for 8 deaths compared with 2.6 expected ($p<0.001$). Three of these were due to HD (0.5 expected). Three were lymphosarcomas and 2 were myelogenous leukemias, 1 acute and 1 chronic. Olin concluded that chemists who continue laboratory work after graduation, especially those working with organic compounds, are at increased risk of death from cancer.

Olin and Ahlbom (86) then expanded the cohort of chemistry graduates from the Royal Institute of Technology to include all male chemists who were graduated between 1930 and 1959. These were followed to assess vital status until the end of 1977. A similar cohort of male architects who were graduated from the same school during the same period of time was also followed. The mortality experience of these two groups of graduates was compared with each other and with that for the general Swedish male population. Both chemists and architects had a lower total mortality than that of the general population. The chemists had a higher mortality from cancer than did the general population or the architects. This higher cancer mortality was primarily due to an excess of lymphoid and hemopoietic neoplasms and brain tumors. Three cases of HD observed (0.7 expected, $p = 0.03$) were among organic chemists. Two cases of myelogenous leukemia (1 chronic), 1 case of lymphosarcoma, and 1 case of reticulum cell sarcoma were also observed among chemists. There were no lymphoid or hemopoietic cancers observed among the architects. The frequency of brain tumors was significantly elevated among chemists in comparison to the general population ($p = 0.01$). There was no tendency for clustering found for the 3 cases of HD. The architects had similar background and living conditions during their years of education but experienced no cases of lymphoid or hemopoietic cancers, although the cohort was small. The authors concluded that the most probable explanation for the high cancer mortality among chemists is their exposure to chemical substances during their education and in their occupation.

Hardell et al. (44) conducted a matched case-control study of malignant lymphoma (HD and NHL) and found that past exposure to phenoxy acids, chlorophenols, and organic solvents was more frequent among cases than controls. The cases consisted of all men aged 25 to 85 years, with histologically verified malignant lymphoma, who were admitted to the Department of Oncology, Umea, Sweden, between 1974 and 1978. Controls for living cases were identified from the Swedish National Population Registry and matched according to gender, age, and place of residence with cases. Controls for deceased cases were extracted from the National Registry of Causes of Death and matched by year of death, gender, age (± 5 years), and place of residence. Self-administered questionnaires of cases, controls, or relatives of the deceased were used to assess exposures. The sample consisted of 60 cases of HD, 109 NHL, and 338 controls. Sixty-two cases and their controls were deceased at the time of the study. The authors concluded that occupational exposure to organic solvents, chlorophenols and/or phenoxy acids constitutes a risk factor for malignant lymphoma, including HD, and suggested the mode of action may be immunologic depression or mutagenic effects.

HODGKIN'S DISEASE

Hodgkin's disease refers to a group of malignancies characterized by the presence of Reed-Sternberg cells in the lymph nodes and other organs. Although HD appears to be due to a peripheral lymphoid lesion and not a stem cell lesion, and thus is less likely to have arisen in the bone marrow, it is included in the group of diseases examined here because it is frequently included in analyses with all lymphomas or with lymphohemopoietic cancers.

Grufferman (38) has reviewed the epidemiology of HD. Although a great deal is known about this disease, and the idea persists that HD may have an infectious origin, its etiology is still unknown. What is known is that environmental factors play an important role. The primary occupational link has been with woodworking, such as among carpenters and sawmill workers. Other occupational groups for which an excess of HD has been reported are teachers, nurses, physicians, and chemists.

Gutensohn and Cole (41) reviewed the epidemiology of HD with particular attention to the evidence relating to an infectious etiology and contagion. Hodgkin's disease has a bimodal age-incidence curve that rises after age 10, peaks in the mid to late 20s, declines until about age 45, and then increases steadily with age. The rates among children were found to decrease and among young adults to increase concurrently with economic development; among older people, the increase of incidence with age is stable during changes in economic development. A variety of studies provided consistent evidence of increased risk of HD among persons of higher social class, particularly among the young. The HD risk for young adults is associated with the social environment during childhood, showing increased risk among persons from small families, with early birth-order positions, and from good living conditions, i.e., factors diminishing and delaying exposure to infectious agents. The authors found that these associations support the hypothesis that HD may be an age-dependent host response to a common infection. However, Gutensohn and Cole found little evidence overall to support the hypothesis that HD is a contagious disease, that is, transmitted by person-to-person contact. They note that the disease may be initiated by an infection but may not be transmissible. The consistent association of HD risk with both elevated Epstein-Barr virus (EBV) titers and history of infectious mononucleosis among diverse populations was found to be noteworthy, but the evidence for EBV as an etiologic agent for HD is still inconclusive.

Regarding the association with occupational exposure to wood, Gutensohn and Cole (41) reviewed five studies (1,36,39,76,92) and concluded that the overall consistency of the association of HD with wood exposure supports its validity. They suggested that chronic wood dust exposure may provide continuing antigenic stimulation, similar to the oncogenic mechanism proposed for virally induced HD, and consistent with the primary role of the macrophage in pathogenesis of the disease.

Olsson and Brandt (88) reported finding an unusually high prevalence of occupations characterized by the handling of chemicals in men with HD. They studied 88 patients between the ages of 20 and 65 years who had been diagnosed and treated for HD during 1973 through 1978 at the Department of Oncology, University Hospital, Lund, Sweden. The case records included information on occupation at diagnosis and histologic classifications. The control patients included 100 men treated for nonmalignant disorders during 1977, 100 treated for allergies during 1977, and 32 men with chronic leukemias seen during 1969 through 1977, all in the age group 20 to 65 years. Occupations indicating a high degree of exposure to chemicals included chemists, painters and sprayers, glass and pottery workers, chemical processing workers, rubber product workers, plastics workers, and photographic laboratory workers. Of the 88 HD patients, 17 had been employed in these occupations, compared with 6 (2% to 3%) among the control group. Moreover, occupational exposure to chemicals was uncommon in HD patients aged 20 to 30 years, whereas in older patients 26% to 32% were occupationally handling chemicals. The authors concluded that occupational exposure to chemical agents may be important in the development of HD in men over age 30. However, they cautioned that occupational titles obtained from case records give insufficient information on occupational hazards.

Benn et al. (14) were unable to confirm the finding of Olsson and Brandt among 558 cases of HD reported to a population-based cancer registry between 1962 to 1976 in the Greater Manchester area of England. They found occupational exposure to chemicals among 3.8% of HD cases, compared with 6.6% of 290 chronic leukemia cases and 3.9% of a group of 33,097 men with other neoplasms for 1972–75. Also, they could not find a more marked association with occupation in those over age 30.

Fonte et al. (33) also could not confirm the findings of Olsson and Brandt in a study in Italy. They found that workers in chemical, pharmaceutical, plastic, and rubber industries were not at increased risk of HD, but did find increased risk of HD among higher socioeconomic groups, teachers and woodworkers, confirming earlier findings.

Despite some indications to the contrary, possibly stemming from imprecise estimations of occupational exposures, evidence seems to be accumulating that occupational factors, including chemical exposures, may play a more important role in the etiology of HD than has been assumed in the past.

DISCUSSION AND CONCLUSIONS

Many additional studies have indicated associations between occupation, possible occupational exposures to chemicals, and increases in the occurrence of various cancers of the lymphoid and hemopoietic systems. These have not been reviewed here because of space and time constraints, but are listed in Table 4 so that the reader may pursue these lines of etiologic evidence more thoroughly.

The main points that may be derived from this review are tempered by the nature of the disease entities, the nature of the populations in which these diseases occur, the nature of the exposures and documentation of those exposures, and the methods used to discover and evaluate relationships between chemical exposure and disease. The diseases are relatively rare and generally occur after a long induction period. At this stage of our understanding, little information is available to differentiate chemical etiologic agents for specific tumor cell types or cells of origin, with the

TABLE 4. *Additional studies of increased risks of lympho/hemopoietic cancers in certain occupations*

Implicated occupation or chemical exposure	Cancer sites	Reference
Aluminum reduction	Lymphoid and hemopoietic	(95)
Anesthetic gases	Lymphoid and reticuloendothelial	(21,22,113)
Asbestos	B-cell neoplasms	(59)
	Large-cell lymphomas	(96)
	Non-Hodgkin's lymphoma	(104,119)
Electrical workers	Leukemia	(67)
Electrical and magnetic fields		(75)
PCBs	Leukemia	(66)
Ethylene oxide:		
Production	Lymphoid and myeloid leukemia	(49)
Production	Hodgkin's disease	(80)
Sterilizing	Acute and chronic myeloid leukemia and microglobulinemia	(48)
Farming	Lymphoid and hemopoietic	(16)
	Non-Hodgkin's lymphoma	(23)
	Lymphoid leukemia	(30)
	Leukemia	(64)
Dairy	Lymphosarcoma; lymphocytic leukemia	(46)
Gold mining	Lymphoid and hemopoietic	(68)
Health-related occupations	Leukemia	(64)
Metal workers:		(34)
Metal mill	Leukemia	
Welders	Hodgkin's disease; multiple myeloma	
Machinists	Multiple myeloma	
Newspaper web pressmen	Leukemia	(91)
Painters in construction industry	Leukemia	(114)
Pentachlorophenol (dioxins?)	Non-Hodgkin's lymphoma (scalp)	(15)
Phenoxy acids & chlorophenols	Lymphoma; Hodgkin's disease	(42–44)
Printing	Leukemia; multiple myeloma; Hodgkin's disease	(37)
Radiation plus		
benzene	Leukemia	(58)
solvents	Leukemia	(32)
Styrene-butadiene rubber	Leukemia	(73)
Styrene-polystyrene	Leukemia; lymphoma; Hodgkin's disease	(83)
Styrene products	Lymphoid leukemia	(89)
Vinyl chloride	Lymphoid and hemopoietic	(50)
Woodworkers	Leukemia	(105)

possible exception of benzene and acute myelogenous leukemia, the most prevalent type of leukemia associated with benzene exposure. Even this is subject to change, as can be seen from the accumulation of studies among benzene-exposed chemical, refinery, and rubber workers, where increases in mortality from lymphatic leukemia, lymphoma, and multiple myeloma have also been observed. It is probable that some combination of exposure level and duration, host factors, and other physical, chemical, or biologic exposures determines the eventual cell type affected by exposure to a chemical such as benzene. Because of the great variety of occupations and processes where benzene has been used, the potential for exposure of large numbers of people in their occupations has existed. This has also permitted the evaluation of risks in many occupations where the primary consistent factor present was benzene. The next step is to determine whether organic solvents are implicated with or without benzene as a contaminant. It may not be possible to make these fine distinctions with human studies where multiple exposures are a fact of life and where one must depend on information derived from experimental studies in nonhuman systems.

Consistent findings such as those reported for occupations with benzene exposure are beginning to appear for other occupations, such as woodworking, where an increased risk of HD has been indicated. The next step is to examine large data bases for several types of woodworking occupations, such as has been done by Stellman and Garfinkel (105), to see if differential disease rates can provide clues to etiologic differences. Exposures to various agents in these diverse woodworking occupations should be defined and compared. Again, a look at the experimental data would be useful to see which of these agents or groups of agents is the most likely causative agent.

Our understanding of the role played by chemical agents in the etiology of human lymphoid and hemopoietic cancers is still in its infancy, but it is being greatly enhanced by the increasing information that has been published in the occupational epidemiologic literature during the past 10 years.

ACKNOWLEDGMENTS

Many thanks to R. P. Nugent, R. D. Irons, R. Moure-Eraso, R. R. Tice, J. G. Dobbins, E. P. Cronkite, and C. Gordon for their thoughtful and helpful comments on the manuscript.

REFERENCES

1. Abramson, J. H., Pridan, H., Sacks, M. I., Avitzour, M., and Peritz, E. (1978): A case-control study of Hodgkin's disease in Israel. *J. Natl. Cancer Inst.*, 61:307–314.
2. Adamson, R. H., and Seiber, S. M. (1981): Chemically induced leukemia in humans. *Environ. Health Perspect.*, 39:93–103.
3. Agu, V. U., Christensen, B. L., and Buffler, P. A. (1980): Geographic patterns of multiple myeloma: Racial and industrial correlates, State of Texas, 1969–71. *J. Natl. Cancer Inst.*, 65:735–738.
4. Aksoy, M. (1977): Leukemia in workers due to occupational exposure to benzene. *New Istanbul Contrib. Clin. Sci.*, 12:3–14.
5. Aksoy, M. (1980): Different types of malignancies due to occupational exposure to benzene: A review of recent observations in Turkey. *Environ. Res.*, 23:181–190.
6. Aksoy, M., Dincol, K., Erdem, S., and Dincol, G. (1972): Acute leukemia due to chronic exposure to benzene. *Am. J. Med.*, 52:160–166.
7. Aksoy, M., Erdem, S., and Dincol, G. (1974): Leukemia in shoe-workers exposed chronically to benzene. *Blood*, 44:837–841.

8. Aksoy, M., Erdem, S., and Dincol, G. (1976): Types of leukemia in chronic benzene poisoning. A study in thirty-four patients. *Acta Haemat.*, 55:65–72.
9. Aksoy, M., Erdem, S., Dincol, K., Hepyuksel, T., and Dincol, G. (1974): Chronic exposure to benzene as a possible contributary etiologic factor in Hodgkin's disease. *Blut*, 28:293–298.
10. Alderson, M. (1980): Cancer mortality in male hairdressers. *J. Epidemiol. Community Health*, 34:182–185.
11. Alderson, M. (1980): Epidemiology of leukemia. *Adv. Cancer Res.*, 31:1–76.
12. Andjelkovic, D., Taulbee, J., and Symons, M. (1976): Mortality experience of a cohort of rubber workers, 1964–1973. *J. Occup. Med.*, 18:387–394.
13. Bader, J. L. (1980): Epidemiology of leukemia and related diseases—Summary. In: *Advances in Comparative Leukemia Research 1979*, edited by D. S. Yohn, B. A. Lapin, and J. R. Blakeslee, pp. 439–442. Elsevier/North-Holland, New York.
14. Benn, R. T., Mangood, A., and Smith, A. (1979): Hodgkin's disease and occupational exposure to chemicals. *Br. Med. J.*, 2:1143.
15. Bishop, C. M., and Jones, A. H. (1981): Non-Hodgkin's lymphoma of the scalp in workers exposed to dioxins (Letter). *Lancet*, 2:369.
16. Blair, A. (1982): Cancer risks associated with agriculture: epidemiologic evidence. In: *Genetic Toxicology. An Agricultural Perspective*, edited by R. A. Fleck and A. Hollaender, pp. 93–111. Plenum Press, New York.
17. Blattner, W. A. (1982): Multiple myeloma and macroglobulinemia. In: *Cancer Epidemiology and Prevention*, edited by D. Schottenfeld and J. F. Fraumeni, Jr., pp. 795–813. W. B. Saunders Co., Philadelphia.
18. Blattner, W. A., Blair, A., and Mason, T. J. (1981): Multiple myeloma in the United States, 1950–1975. *Cancer*, 48:2547–2554.
19. Brandt, L., Nillson, P. G., and Mitelman, F. (1978): Occupational exposure to petroleum products in men with acute non-lymphocytic leukaemia. *Br. Med. J.*, 1:553.
20. Brown, S. M. (1975): Leukemia and potential benzene exposure. Letter to the editor. *J. Occup. Med.*, 17:5–6.
21. Bruce, D. L., Eide, K. A., Linde, H. W., and Eckenhoff, J. E. (1968): Causes of death among anesthesiologists: a 20-year survey. *Anesthesiology*, 29:565–569.
22. Bruce, D. L., Eide, K. A., Smith, N. J., Seltzer, F., and Dykes, M. H. M. (1974): A prospective survey of anesthesiologist mortality, 1967–1971. *Anesthesiology*, 41:71–74.
23. Cantor, K. P. (1982): Farming and mortality from non-Hodgkin's lymphoma: A case-control study. *Int. J. Cancer*, 29:239–247.
24. Checkoway, H., Wilcosky, T., Wolf, P., and Tyroler, H. (1984): An evaluation of the associations of leukemia and rubber industry solvent exposures. *Am. J. Ind. Med.*, 5:239–249.
25. Cronkite, E. P. (1961): Evidence for radiation and chemicals as leukemogenic agents. *Arch. Environ. Health*, 3:297–303.
26. Cutler, S. J., and Young, J. L., Jr., editors (1975): *Third National Cancer Survey: Incidence Data*. National Cancer Institute Monograph 41. DHEW Publ. No. (NIH) 75-787.
27. Decoufle, P. (1984): Letter to Dr. Peter Infante, Occupational Safety and Health Administration. January 26, 1984.
28. Decoufle, P., Blattner, W., and Blair, A. (1983): Mortality among chemical workers exposed to benzene and other agents. *Environ. Res.*, 30:16–25.
29. Delzell, E., and Monson, R. R. (1982): Mortality among rubber workers: V. Processing workers. *J. Occup. Med.*, 24:539–545.
30. Donham, K. J., Berg, J. W., and Sawin, R. S. (1980): Epidemiologic relationships of the bovine population and human leukemia in Iowa. *Am. J. Epidemiol.*, 112:80–92.
31. Enterline, P. (1979): Lymphomas and benzene. Letter to the editor. *Lancet*, 2:1021.
32. Flodin, U., Andersson, L., Anjou, C.-G., Palm, U.-B., Vikrot, O., and Axelson, O. (1981): A case-referent study on acute myeloid leukemia, background radiation and exposure to solvents and other agents. *Scand. J. Work Environ. Health*, 7:169–178.
33. Fonte, R., Grigis, L., Grigis, P., and Franco, G. (1982): Chemicals and Hodgkin's disease. *Lancet*, 2:50.
34. Gallagher, R. P., and Threlfall, W. J. (1983): Cancer mortality in metal workers. *Can. Med. Assoc. J.*, 129:1191–1194.
35. Greene, M. H. (1982): Non-Hodgkin's lymphoma and mycosis fungoides. In: *Cancer Epidemiology*

and Prevention, edited by D. Schottenfeld and J. F. Fraumeni, Jr., pp. 754–778. W. B. Saunders Co., Philadelphia.

36. Greene, M. H., Brinton, L. A., Fraumeni, J. F., and D'Amico, R. (1978): Familial and sporadic Hodgkin's disease associated with occupational wood exposure. *Lancet*, 2:626–627.

37. Greene, M. H., Hoover, R. N., Eck, R. L., and Fraumeni, J. F., Jr. (1979): Cancer mortality among printing plant workers. *Environ. Res.*, 20:66–73.

38. Grufferman, S. (1982): Hodgkin's disease. In: *Cancer Epidemiology and Prevention*, edited by D. Schottenfeld and J. F. Fraumeni, Jr., pp. 739–753. W. B. Saunders Co., Philadelphia.

39. Grufferman, S., Duong, T., and Cole, P. (1976): Occupation and Hodgkin's disease. *J. Natl. Cancer Inst.*, 57:1193–1195.

40. Guidotti, S., Wright, W. E., and Peters, J. M. (1982): Multiple myeloma in cosmetologists. *Am. J. Ind. Med.*, 3:169–171.

41. Gutensohn, N., and Cole, P. (1980): Epidemiology of Hodgkin's disease. *Semin. Oncol.*, 7:92–102.

42. Hardell, L., and Axelson, O. (1982): Soft-tissue sarcoma, malignant lymphoma, and exposure to phenoxyacids or chlorophenols. *Lancet*, 1:1408–1409.

43. Hardell, L., and Bengtsson, N. O. (1983): Epidemiological study of socioeconomic factors and clinical findings in Hodgkin's disease, and reanalysis of previous data regarding chemical exposure. *Br. J. Cancer*, 48:217–225.

44. Hardell, L., Eriksson, M., Lenner, P., and Lundgren, E. (1981): Malignant lymphoma and exposure to chemicals, especially organic solvents, chlorophenols and phenoxy acids: a case-control study. *Br. J. Cancer*, 43:169–176.

45. Harrington, J. M., and Shannon, H.S. (1975): Mortality study of pathologists and medical laboratory technicians. *Br. Med. J.*, 4:329–332.

46. Heath, C. W., Jr. (1970): Human leukemia: Genetic and environmental clusters. *Comp. Leuk. Res. Bibl. Haematologica*, 36:649–653.

47. Heath, C. W., Jr. (1982): The leukemias. In: *Cancer Epidemiology and Prevention*, edited by D. Schottenfeld and J. F. Fraumeni, Jr., Chapter 41, pp. 728–738. W. B. Saunders Co., Philadelphia.

48. Hogstedt, C., Malmqvist, N., and Wadman, B. (1979): Leukemia in workers exposed to ethylene oxide. *JAMA*, 241:1132–1133.

49. Hogstedt, C., Rohlen, O., Berndtsson, B. S., Axelson, O., and Ehrenberg, L. (1979): A cohort study of mortality and cancer incidence in ethylene oxide production workers. *Br. J. Ind. Med.*, 36:276–280.

50. Infante, P. F. (1981): Observations of the site-specific carcinogenicity of vinyl chloride to humans. *Environ. Health Perspect.*, 41:89–94.

51. Infante, P. F. (1982): General discussion. J. W. Lloyd, moderator. In: *Brain Tumors in the Chemical Industry*, edited by I. J. Selikoff and E. C. Hammond. *Ann. NY Acad. Sci.*, 381:184.

52. Infante, P. F., Rinsky, R. A., Wagoner, J. K., and Young, R. J. (1977): Leukaemia in benzene workers. *Lancet*, 2:76–78.

53. Infante, P. F., Rinsky, R. A., Wagoner, J. K., and Young, R. J. (1977): Benzene and leukemia (Letter). *Lancet*, 2:868–869.

54. Infante, P. F., and White, M. C. (1983): Benzene: Epidemiologic observations of leukemia by cell type and adverse health effects associated with low-level exposure. *Environ. Health Perspect.*, 52:75–82.

55. Infante, P. F., White, M. C., and Chu, K. C. (1984): Assessment of leukemia mortality associated with occupational exposure to benzene (Letter). *Risk Analysis*, 4:9–13.

56. International Agency for Research on Cancer (IARC) (1982): *IARC Monographs on the Evaluation of the Carcinogenic Risk of Chemicals to Humans. The Rubber Industry*, Vol. 28. IARC, Lyon, France.

57. International Agency for Research on Cancer (IARC) (1982): *IARC Monographs on the Evaluation of the Carcinogenic Risk of Chemicals to Humans. Some Industrial Chemicals and Dyestuffs*, Vol. 29. IARC, Lyon, France.

58. Ishimaru, T., Okada, H., Tomiyasu, T., Tsuchimoto, T., Hoshino, T., and Ichimaru, M. (1971): Occupational factors in the epidemiology of leukemia in Hiroshima and Nagasaki. *Am. J. Epidemiol.*, 93:157–165.

59. Kagan, E., Jacobson, R. J., Yeung, K., and Haidak, D. J. (1979): Asbestos-associated neoplasms of B cell lineage. *Am. J. Med.*, 67:325–330.

60. Kilpikari, I. (1982): Mortality among male rubber workers in Finland. *Arch. Environ. Health*, 37:295–299.
61. Kilpikari, I., Pukkala, E., Lehtonen, M., and Hakama, M. (1982): Cancer incidence among Finnish rubber workers. *Int. Arch. Occup. Environ. Health*, 51:65–71.
62. Lemen, R. (1982): General discussion. J. W. Lloyd, moderator. In: *Brain Tumors in the Chemical Industry*, edited by I. J. Selikoff and E. C. Hammond. *Ann. NY Acad. Sci.*, 381:182.
63. Li, F. P., Fraumeni, J. F., Jr., Mantel, N., and Miller, R. W. (1969): Cancer mortality among chemists. *J. Nat. Cancer Inst.*, 43:1159–1164.
64. Linos, A., Kyle, R. A., O'Fallon, W. M., and Kurland, L. T. (1980): A case-control study of occupational exposures and leukaemia. *Int. J. Epidemiol.*, 9:131–135.
65. Mack, T. M., and Preston-Martin, S. (1980): Trends in the epidemiology of the leukemias and lymphomas. In: *Advances in Comparative Leukemia Research 1979*, edited by D. S. Yohn, B. A. Lapin, and J. R. Blakeslee, pp. 431–438. Elsevier/North-Holland, New York.
66. Maroni, M., Colombi, A., Arbosti, G., Cantoni, S., and Foa, V. (1981): Occupational exposure to polychlorinated biphenyls in electrical workers. II Health effects. *Br. J. Ind. Med.*, 38:55–60.
67. McDowall, M. E. (1983): Leukaemia mortality in electrical workers in England and Wales. *Lancet*, 1:246.
68. McGlashan, N. D., Harington, J. S., and Bradshaw, E. (1982): Eleven sites of cancer in black gold miners from southern Africa: A geographic enquiry. *Br. J. Cancer*, 46:947–954.
69. McMichael, A. J., Andjelkovic, D. A., and Tyroler, H. A. (1976): Cancer mortality among rubber workers: An epidemiologic study. *Ann. NY Acad. Sci.*, 271:125–137.
70. McMichael, A. J., Spirtas, R., Gamble, J. F., and Tousey, P. M. (1976): Mortality among rubber workers: Relationship to specific jobs. *J. Occup. Med.*, 18:178–185.
71. McMichael, A. J., Spirtas, R., and Kupper, L. L. (1974): An epidemiologic study of mortality within a cohort of rubber workers, 1964–72. *J. Occup. Med.*, 16:458–464.
72. McMichael, A. J., Spirtas, R., Kupper, L. L., and Gamble, J. F. (1975): Solvent exposure and leukemia among rubber workers: An epidemiologic study. *J. Occup. Med.*, 17:234–239.
73. Meinhardt, T. J., Lemen, R. A., Crandall, M. S., and Young, R. J. (1982): Environmental epidemiologic investigation of the styrene-butadiene rubber industry. Mortality patterns with discussion of the hematopoietic and lymphatic malignancies. *Scand. J. Work Environ. Health*, 8:250–259.
74. Milham, S., Jr. (1976): *Occupational Mortality in Washington State, 1950–1971*, Volume I. HEW Publ. No. (NIOSH) 76-175-A, NIOSH, Cincinnati, Ohio.
75. Milham, S., Jr. (1982): Mortality from leukemia in workers exposed to electrical and magnetic fields. *N. Engl. J. Med.*, 307:249.
76. Milham, S., Jr., and Hesser, J. E. (1967): Hodgkin's disease in woodworkers. *Lancet*, 2:136–137.
77. Monson, R. J. (1980): *Occupational Epidemiology*. CRC Press Inc., Boca Raton, Fl.
78. Monson, R. R., and Fine, L. J. (1978): Cancer mortality and morbidity among rubber workers. *J. Natl. Cancer Inst.*, 61:1047–1053.
79. Monson, R. R., and Nakano, K. K. (1976): Mortality among rubber workers I. White male union employees in Akron, Ohio. *Am. J. Epidemiol.*, 103:284–296.
80. Morgan, R. W., Claxton, K. W., Divine, B. J., Kaplan, S. D., and Harris, V. B. (1981): Mortality among ethylene oxide workers. *J. Occup. Med.*, 23:767–770.
81. Morgan, T. W., and Banks, P. M. (1983): Histopathology of malignant lymphomas. In: *Hematology*, 3rd ed., edited by W. J. Williams, E. Beutler, A. J. Erslev, and M. A. Lichtman, Chapter 117, pp. 1003–1011. McGraw Hill, New York.
82. Moure, R. (1982): General discussion. J. W. Lloyd, moderator. In: *Brain Tumors in the Chemical Industry*, edited by I. J. Selikoff and E. C. Hammond. *Ann. NY Acad. Sci.*, 381:181–182.
83. Nicholson, W. J., Selikoff, I. J., and Seidman, H. (1978): Mortality experience of styrene-polystyrene polymerization workers. *Scand. J. Work Environ. Health*, 4[Suppl.] 2:247–252.
84. O'Conor, G. T. (1984): Geography of lymphoid neoplasia: An overview. In: *Pathogenesis of Leukemias and Lymphomas: Environmental Influences*, edited by I. T. Magrath, G. T. O'Conor, and B. Ramot, pp. 1–8. Raven Press, New York.
85. Olin, G. R. (1978): The hazards of a chemical laboratory environment—a study of the mortality in two cohorts of Swedish chemists. *Am. Ind. Hyg. Assoc. J.*, 39:557–562.
86. Olin, G. R., and Ahlbom, A. (1980): The cancer mortality among Swedish chemists graduated during three decades. *Environ. Res.*, 22:154–169.

87. Olin, R. (1976): Leukaemia and Hodgkin's disease among Swedish chemistry graduates. *Lancet*, 2:916.
88. Olsson, H., and Brandt, L. (1979): Occupational handling of chemicals preceding Hodgkin's disease in men. *Br. Med. J.*, 2:580–581.
89. Ott, M. G., Kolesar, R. C., Scharnweber, H. C., Schneider, E. J., and Venable, J. R. (1980): A mortality survey of employees engaged in the development or manufacture of styrene-based products. *J. Occup. Med.*, 22:445–460.
90. Ott, M. G., Townsend, J. C., Fishbeck, W. A., and Langner, R. A. (1978): Mortality among indivduals occupationally exposed to benzene. *Arch. Environ. Health*, 33:3–10.
91. Paganini-Hill, A., Glazer, E., Henderson, B. E., and Ross, R. K. (1980): Cause-specific mortality among newspaper web pressmen. *J. Occup. Med.*, 22:542–544.
92. Petersen, G. R., and Milham, S., Jr. (1974): Brief communication: Hodgkin's disease mortality and occupational exposure to wood. *J. Natl. Cancer Inst.*, 53:957–958.
93. Riggan, W. B., Van Bruggen, J., Acquavella, J. F., Beaubier, J., and Mason, T. J. (1983): *U.S. Cancer Mortality Rates and Trends, 1950–1979*. 3 Volumes. National Cancer Institute/ U.S. Environmental Protection Agency, EPA 600/1-83-015. U.S. Government Printing Office, Washington, D.C.
94. Rinsky, R. A., Young, R. J., and Smith, A. B. (1981): Leukemia in benzene workers. *Am. J. Ind. Med.*, 2:217–245.
95. Rockette, H. E., and Arena, V. C. (1983): Mortality studies of aluminum reduction plant workers: potroom and carbon department. *J. Occup. Med.*, 25:549–557.
96. Ross, R., Dworsky, R., Nichols, P., Paganini-Hill, A., Wright, W., Koss, M., Lukes, R., and Henderson, B. (1982): Asbestos exposure and lymphomas of the gastrointestinal tract and oral cavity. *Lancet*, 2:1118–1119.
97. Rundles, R. W. (1983): Chronic lymphocytic leukemia. In: *Hematology*, 3rd ed., edited by W. J. Williams, E. Beutler, A. J. Erslev, and M. A., Lichtman, pp. 981–998. McGraw Hill, New York.
98. Rushton, L., and Alderson, M. R. (1981): A case-control study to investigate the association between exposure to benzene and deaths from leukemia in oil refinery workers. *Br. J. Cancer*, 43:77–83.
99. Schimpff, S. C., Schimpff, C. R., Brager, D. M., and Wiernik, P. H. (1975): Leukemia and lymphoma patients interlinked by prior social contact. *Lancet*, 1:124–129.
100. Schottenfeld, D., and Haas, J. F. (1981): Carcinogens in the workplace. In: *Cancer Causing Chemicals*, edited by N. I. Sax, pp. 14–27. Van Nostrand Reinhold, New York.
101. Schottenfeld, D., Warshauer, M. E., Zauber, A. G., Meikle, J. G., and Hart, B. R. (1981): A prospective study of morbidity and mortality in petroleum industry employees in the United States—A preliminary report. In: *Quantification of Occupational Cancer*, edited by R. Peto and M. Schneiderman, pp. 247–260. Banbury Report 9, Cold Spring Harbor Laboratory, New York.
102. Searle, C. E., Waterhouse, J. A. H., Henman, B. A., Bartlett, D., and McCombie, S. (1978): Epidemiological study of the mortality of British chemists. *Br. J. Cancer*, 38:192–193.
103. Smith, P. R., and Lickiss, J. N. (1980): Benzene and lymphomas (Letter). *Lancet*, 1:719.
104. Spanedda, R., Barbieri, D., and LaCorte, R. (1983): Asbestos and non-Hodgkin's lymphoma. Letter to the editor. *Lancet*, 1:190.
105. Stellman, S. D., and Garfinkel, L. (1984): Cancer mortality among woodworkers. *Am. J. Ind. Med.*, 5:343–357.
106. Tabershaw, I. R., and Lamm, S. H. (1977): Benzene and leukemia (Letter). *Lancet*, 2:867–868.
107. Thomas, T. L., Decoufle, P., and Moure-Eraso, R. (1980): Mortality among workers employed in petroleum refining and petrochemical plants. *J. Occup. Med.*, 22:97–103.
108. Thomas, T. L., Waxweiler, R. J., Crandall, M. S., White, D. W., Moure-Eraso, R., and Fraumeni, J. F., Jr. (1984): Cancer mortality patterns by work category in three Texas oil refineries. *Am. J. Ind. Med.*, 6:3–16.
109. Thomas, T. L., Waxweiler, R. J., Moure-Eraso, R., Itaya, S., and Fraumeni, J. F., Jr. (1982): Mortality patterns among workers in three Texas oil refineries. *J. Occup. Med.*, 24:135–41.
110. Thorpe, J. J. (1974): Epidemiologic survey of leukemia in persons potentially exposed to benzene. *J. Occup. Med.*, 16:375–382.
111. Tsai, S. P., Wen, C. P., Weiss, N. S., Wong, O., McClellan, W. A., and Gibson, R. L. (1983): Retrospective mortality and medical surveillance studies of workers in benzene areas of refineries. *J. Occup. Med.*, 25:685–692.

112. Tyroler, H. A., Andjelkovic, D., Harris, R., Lednar, W., McMichael, A., and Symons, M. (1976): Chronic diseases in the rubber industry. *Environ. Health Perspect.*, 17:13–20.
113. Vessey, M. P. (1978): Epidemiological studies of the occupational hazards of anaesthesia. A review. *Anaesthesia*, 33:430–438.
114. Viadana, E., and Bross, I. D. J. (1972): Leukemia and occupations. *Prev. Med.*, 1:513–521.
115. Vianna, N. J., and Polan, A. (1979): Lymphomas and occupational benzene exposure. *Lancet*, 1:1394–1395.
116. Vigliani, E. C. (1976): Leukemia associated with benzene exposure. *Ann. NY Acad. Sci.*, 271:143–151.
117. Vigliani, E. C., and Forni, A. (1976): Benzene and leukemia. *Environ. Res.*, 11:122–127.
118. Vigliani, E. C., and Saita, G. (1964): Benzene and leukemia. *N. Engl. J. Med.*, 271:872–876.
119. Waxweiler, R. J., and Robinson, C. (1983): Asbestos and non-Hodgkin's lymphoma. Letter to the editor. *Lancet*, 1:189–190.
120. Wen, C. P., Tsai, S. P., McClellan, W. A., and Gibson, R. L. (1983): Long-term mortality study of oil refinery workers I. Mortality of hourly and salaried workers. *Am. J. Epidemiol.*, 118:526–542.
121. World Health Organization (1976): *ICD-0, International Classification of Diseases for Oncology.* W.H.O., Geneva.
122. World Health Organization (1977): *Manual of the International Statistical Classification of Diseases, Injuries, and Causes of Death.* W.H.O., Geneva.

Subject Index